PLANT BASED
NUTRITION
for
LIFE

a recipe and resource guide

Real Food for Healthy People

A Resource Guide for Whole Food Plant Based Cooking

Distributed in the United States by Ingram Sparks, 1 Ingram Boulevard, La Vergne TN

Hardcover ISBN 9780692582701

eBook ISBN 9780692593462

www.foodnotmeds.com

info@foodnotmeds.com

PRINTED IN THE UNITED STATES OF AMERICA

Introduction

The Concept Behind Real Food

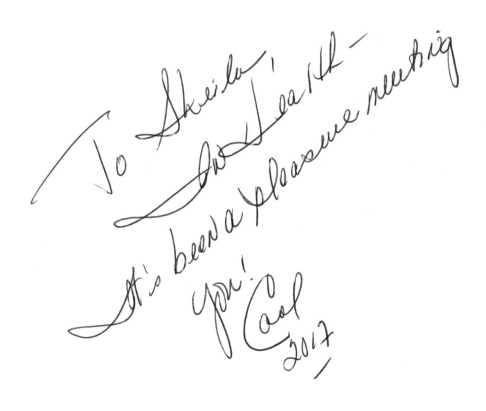

To Sheila,
Good Health —
It's been a pleasure meeting
you! Carl
2017

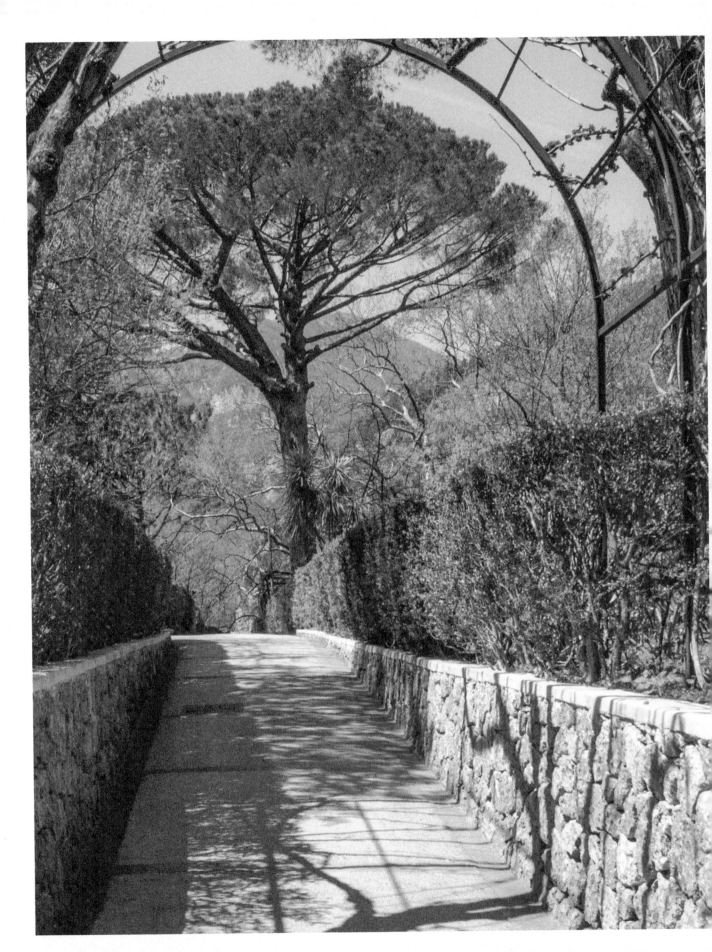

"Somewhere close behind the need for air and water is the need for food."

-L.J. Martin

How well that describes the point I was at several years ago when I was in need of food... and not just any food, but food that would keep me healthy. I knew inherently that the food I was eating wasn't going to keep me healthy much longer and I knew I was nutrition deprived.

Although I was raised on a typical Mediterranean Diet, it had become far too rich in my adult life with heavy cheeses, desserts and large portion sizes of food. I loved to cook and I was good at it, but I had reached a stage in my life where I had concerns about creeping cholesterol and blood pressure numbers. My suspicions were confirmed while sitting in a doctor's office in 2006 and hearing a suggestion that I take cholesterol-lowering medication. As someone who resists even taking an aspirin and has always been opposed to altering my biochemistry with medications, it was a frightening moment and the impetus for change.

But, change, how? What did I really need? It felt strangely odd to me that I didn't have the answers despite the fact that I had formal undergraduate academic training in biochemistry and biology and I had a graduate degree in clinical nutrition. It took a while and then it clicked, "clinical nutrition" is just that, clinical, for people with acute and chronic diagnoses. I was looking for *preventative* nutrition, a different kind of answer.

Don't get me wrong here; I'm happy to have the background that I do. It allows me to read a research paper and discern if a study is worthy of merit, and it allows me to understand the body's chemical processes, our anatomy, how digestion works and a myriad of other things. It was all a great basis for beginning my search but it didn't provide the answer to what I was seeking despite looking everywhere. I needed to find answers for myself and for my clients who I began noticing were increasingly coming to me wanting to get off medications due to their side effects. I saw more and more of what I began calling the "holy trinity" of commonly prescribed drugs: cholesterol lowering, blood pressure lowering and diabetes medications. It seemed that once that path was taken it was almost impossible to eliminate their continued usage.

Frustrated, but resolved to find an answer, I signed up for a year long online course in nutrition that provided me an overview of all the dietary theories in place today. Guess what? There are over 100 of them. After close scrutiny I could tell which made sense to me and which I wouldn't even consider as an option for developing and maintaining good health.

After the initial year of study, research and comparisons, I knew what I wanted and needed: a diet preventing the chronic diseases we suffer from today such as heart disease, diabetes and cancer. That diet needed to be rich in antioxidants which would combat inflammation, one of the underlying causes of all chronic disease and a diet without high levels of saturated fat, sugar and white flour. It had to be one that eliminates processed foods, virtually anything pre-packaged and invariably those encased in a crinkly wrapper.

My reasons for this? Well, regardless of how confusing the news articles can be about nutrition, one thing is for sure – refined white sugar is deadly and we eat plenty of it. Let's be honest and call it a drug rather than food. And despite what the New York Times tells us, the average American should be eating less saturated fat that comes from meat and dairy if they want to avoid a myriad of problems. There is plenty of research over the last 20 years for that solid conclusion. Fat from these sources raises LDL cholesterol and when LDL cholesterol gets oxidized in our arteries it causes plaque. When the protective cap on plaque in our arteries ruptures it releases a clot(s) causing heart attacks and strokes. Someone dies of a heart attack or a stroke every minute in the U.S. Reducing animal sources of saturated fat and replacing it with carbohydrates from fruits and vegetables (not refined carbohydrates originating from white sugar and flour) has significantly positive health benefits.

Although I was never a "junk food eater" and I made just about everything from "scratch," I decided to get hyper-vigilant about eliminating the chemicals added to boxed and processed food. I became deeply concerned about the toxins we take in each day overloading our liver (which has to detoxify our blood) by removing harmful toxins. We are exposed to so many unavoidable toxins from our environment that we don't need to add additional ones in food. I decided to buy foods without a label and to focus mainly on organically grown fruits, vegetables, herbs and grains, all delivering the powerful phytochemicals that we need daily. This all seemed like a tall order, especially paired with not wanting to eat anything with GMO's, refined sugars of any kind or anything with refined white flour. It sounds daunting but what it all really "boils down" to is a whole food plant based diet. Now I had something to work with and I was excited!

Armed with the academic learning and a year of my own research identifying real food for a healthy life, I headed to the bookstore to get guidance and recipes needed to start this new eating plan. Wow, was I in for a surprise. I stood in front of four aisles packed with cookbooks hardly knowing where to start. I was undaunted in my efforts and many titles caught my interest.

I found Vegetarian cookbooks with recipes loaded with sugar and fat, Vegan cookbooks loaded with oil and salt, Plant Based cookbooks with recipes that were bland and tasteless, and Mediterranean cookbooks loaded with cheeses, meats and foods that I knew were going to sabotage my efforts by eating them. I found a few good ones that could be adapted but over time I probably bought 50 books trying to combine a recipe here and there to get a full complement of what I was seeking. After a few months of trying this process I brought them all to Half Price Books in the city where I live for re-sale.

Something else was happening at the same time that I was hunting for recipes; I found myself talking to my clients about a real "food only" approach to preventing and reversing chronic illness. Curiously they began asking me for recipes requested that I teach them the culinary skills needed for this type of eating. Simply put, they were telling me they could see the benefits of what I was teaching them, but they didn't know where to start and I couldn't refer them to 50 different cookbooks for answers.

I quickly realized if I was going to give my clients advice to eat "real food for a healthy life," they were going to need some help getting started and the food had to delicious tasting, easy to prepare, satiating, healthful and provide variety so it wouldn't get boring. Wow, what a task I had set up for myself. I was spending countless hours in my "test kitchen" at home developing new recipes, some from "scratch" and others that I converted from my own former favorites. Although I wouldn't call myself a chef, I've had culinary training both in the U.S. and Italy providing a solid foundation for culinary arts and trying new approaches to cooking and baking. I also come from a family of great cooks and I spent a lot of time in the kitchen watching my mother. Surprisingly, what I found most helpful in this quest was my background in biochemistry! I knew what ingredients to combine to make a batter rise, to thicken a sauce and I had the confidence to try new and sometimes unusual flours and spices because I could almost see the chemical reactions they would produce to make a tasty and appealing recipe.

Recipes started developing quickly and as my exposure to the people who wanted "real food for a healthy life" grew, so did their desire for recipes. As a service to my clients and others who were interested, I started offering cooking classes at my home, in the community and at a hospital working with a cardiologist who is proposing real food for his patients. I named my school "The Academy of Plant Based Nutrition and Cooking" and offered classes on a regular basis from May through October, keeping them to the warmer time of the year because we have a lovely outdoor kitchen which my students love. Classes were always filled and attendees consistently became inspired and more confident about incorporating this type of cooking for themselves and their families.

Repeated requests for recipes, the need for creativity and variety and a desire for meals which were not only healthful, but delicious have collectively led to the creation of this cookbook and research guide. Every recipe is solely plant based, is unprocessed, does not contain oil (although a small amount of oil is mentioned as an option if preferred) and is almost 100% gluten free – not an easy task while making food taste good but trying these is believing that it can be done. I'm delighted that you have picked up this book but am even happier about the benefits you will experience because good health really does begin in the kitchen.

If you are new to plant based nutrition, the information provided will save months of trials and error. If you are already on this journey you will surely find some interesting additions to your current repertoire of information and recipes.

I wish you the best in your journey toward optimum health!

Contents

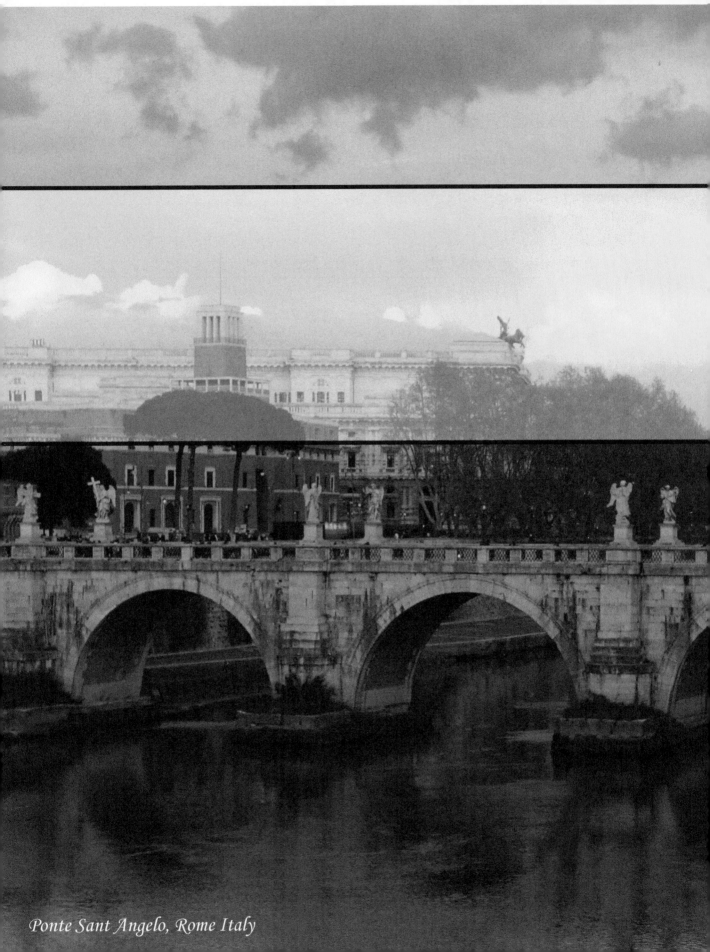

Ponte Sant Angelo, Rome Italy

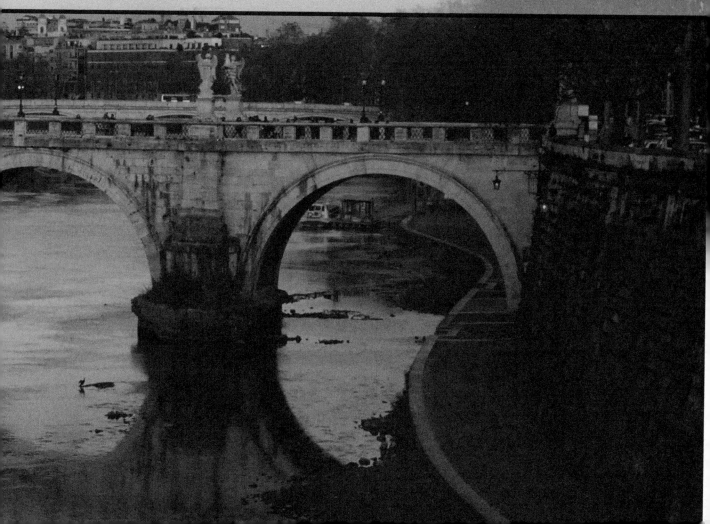

Chapter 1

Preparing for a Successful Outcome

Preparing for a Successful Outcome

The preparation of "real" foods requires some good tools making your life easier in the kitchen and assuring a great outcome. Having the right equipment in the kitchen requires a bit of an investment but it's an investment in good health because good health really does begin in the kitchen. There is no substitute for good quality tools.

Knives: You don't need to go out and buy an 18 piece knife set but having three good knives that fit your hand and can be kept sharp will make your life easier and your prospects for success higher.

Chef's Knife - This knife comes in 8", 9" or 10" sizes. You may prefer a shorter or longer size. It's up to you and what feels more comfortable in your hand. It's the knife that will get the most use, so be willing to spend a little more for it and keep it sharp with a sharpening stone or rod.

Paring Knife - This is a small knife that's used for trimming and other detail work. A 3" or 3½" blade will probably work for most cooks,

Serrated Long Knife - You may use this one the least but it's handy to have for larger vegetables and finished recipes requiring longer slices of food.

Pans:

Heavy bottom pans made of good stainless steel are essential because they distribute heat evenly. You cannot get the same outcome with an aluminum (which should never be used because aluminum gets soft and can get in your food) or other cheap pans. I use pans made of 18/10 (18% stainless steel, 10% nickel) and they cook beautifully. My students sometimes comment that they never get the same results with recipes using their pans - another testament to good quality pans that are heavy enough to distribute heat evenly.

As cooking without oil becomes more popular there are a lot more non-stick pans available. Stay away from Teflon which is toxic and gets in your food. Good non-stick pans are made of ceramic, silica and ceramic/titanium. I have three heavy non-stick grill pans that I use on the stovetop in the winter for grilling vegetables. There's more about grilling vegetables in the next chapter.

Food Processor - Before changing to a whole food plant based diet I only used my food processor for making desserts or chopping large amounts of food. Today it's a staple of the kitchen and I use it for everything from chopping, processing, making nut butters, soups, flour and a million other things. You will read about the many uses for the food processor in the recipes that follow. Many brands exist in the marketplace and they range in price. I use a Cuisinart that costs around $150. A Vita Mix is also very nice to have but if you want to keep your initial costs down stick with a food processor only.

Small Vegetable Peeler - An indispensable little tool allowing you to not only quickly peel carrots and potatoes but can be used as a "finishing tool" making carrot curls or zucchini strips along with many other uses.

Microplane - Used to prepare the "zest" of lemons and oranges (organic to avoid pesticides in food, especially since these are the skins) and can also be used to grate garlic. You may want to buy and use a separate microplane for dedicated use with garlic.

Parchment Paper - Lining all baking and roasting pans with parchment paper eliminates all need for oil and other fats on the pan and produces a wonderful clean, non-stick surface. Watch the labels on parchment paper however. Some may have additives in the paper that get on your food.

Mixing Bowls - At minimum a small, medium and large bowl made of glass or stainless steel.

To start, these are essential. Over time you will undoubtedly want to add more kitchen equipment and tools but you don't need much else to begin making great tasting and healthful meals.

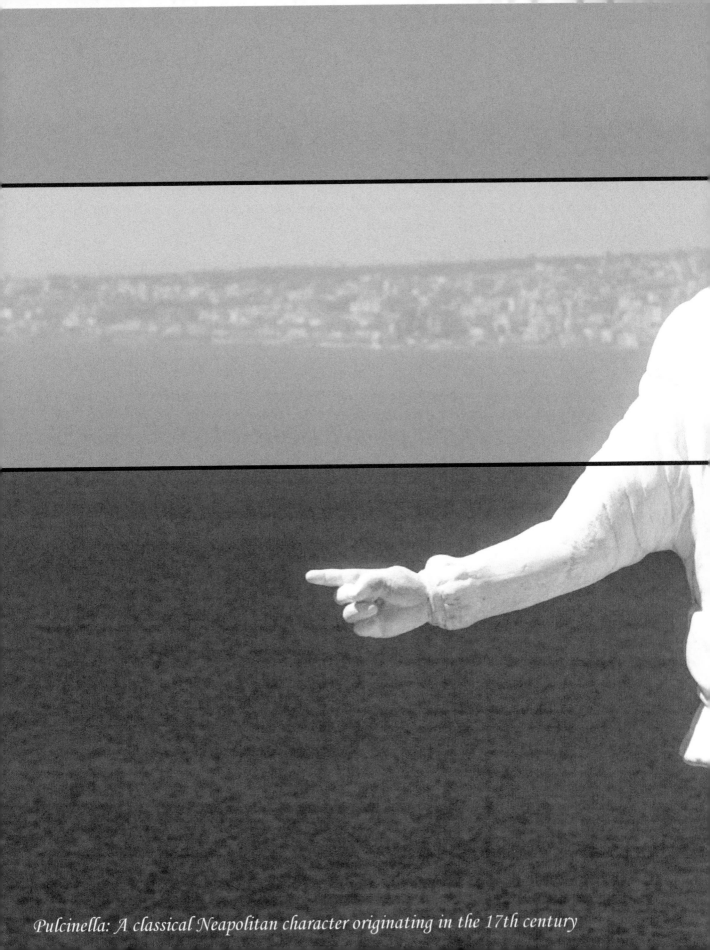

Pulcinella: A classical Neapolitan character originating in the 17th century

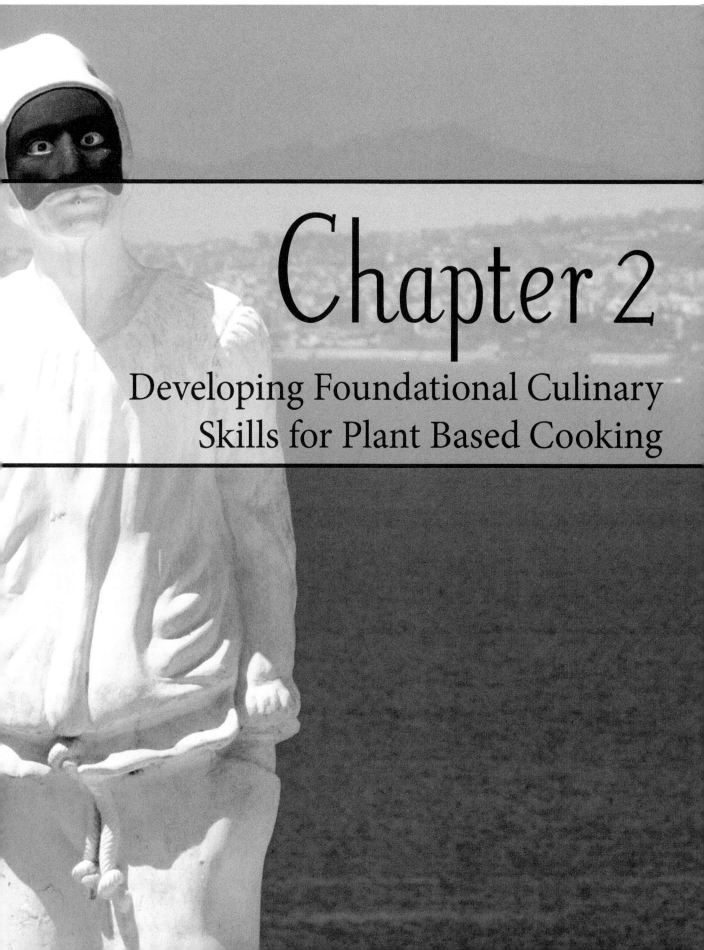

Chapter 2

Developing Foundational Culinary Skills for Plant Based Cooking

Developing Foundational Culinary Skills for "Real Food" Cooking

You don't have to be a professional chef to make wonderful meals for yourself and your family and friends, but a few skills will go far for developing great dishes.

Learning how to cook without oil (or minimal oil) is usually a challenge for most people. Almost every recipe we see calls for oil for frying, baking, drizzling or some other use. When you master the technique for cooking without oil you'll experience the real taste of the foods you are preparing. The key to "no oil technique" is starting with a hot pan. Chapter one covers the type of pan to use: heavy bottom stainless steel or non-stick pan that does not use Teflon.

A test of "readiness" of the pan is to put a couple drops of water on the surface. When the water beads up the pan is ready for cooking. Add your sliced onions, mushrooms or whatever ingredients you are using. Let the heat quickly begin the cooking process then lower the temperature, continue cooking and let the natural sugars and flavors release. If you do need liquid add vegetable stock - either a broth you have prepared in your kitchen (recipe to follow) or a commercially prepared stock. I have used Kitchen Basics brand for years. It's the lowest sodium stock on the market.

Using lemons - A staple of the kitchen is the lemon. You will find lemons to be one of the most frequently used and versatile ingredient in a host of recipes. The juice of a lemon can act as a tenderizer for vegetables, for example, or it can act as a seasoning adding a pop of flavor to almost any dish. The outer skin of the lemon or the zest, adds flavor beyond belief to main dishes and desserts. You can even grill lemon slices and adding intensity and contrast to recipes.

Grilling (and roasting) vegetables - Once you can properly grill and/or roast vegetables with caramelized natural sugars and intensified its natural flavors you have the foundation for a myriad of wonderful dishes. It does take a little technique and a little learning. Fortunately I finally learned how to do it at a cooking class in Italy and I always request vegetable grilling as part of the class when I take groups to Italy. The detail about grilling and roasting will follow in this book.

Making soup stock - A good soup stock is another of those basics that you'll use for sautéing vegetables and for soups, either hearty winter soups or delicate spring asparagus soup. It's simple to do but takes a little time and planning if you are stretched for time.

Using spices - Cooking with real food doesn't rely on salt for flavor but rather uses spices and herbs for both flavor and health reasons. Spices add depth, taste and excitement to dishes that would otherwise be bland. The addition of spices adds rich notes of earthy, smoky, musky, pungent, bitter, sour, sweet to recipes. You'll experiment with a few spices in the recipes that follow. Just adding salt and pepper to recipes seems boring after you've worked with spices. An added benefit is the powerful anti-inflammatory benefits that are yours through the use of spices.

Use of vinegars - Liberal use of spices is followed by the liberal use of vinegars not just any vinegar but the best aged vinegar you can find and additionally, the best vinegars that are aged with fruits and spices. A "topper" of Sicilian lemon, sour apple, blackberry, ginger or champagne vinegar makes all the difference between ordinary and spectacular dishes.

Grilling Vegetables

Grilling vegetables at home is an art. Don't let anyone tell you that you just slice, put them on the grill or in the oven for 3 minutes and you're done. There is more to it.

When you master the art of grilling vegetables you will have the basics of many dishes whether you use the grilled vegetables as a side dish, tossed pasta, used in wraps or as a meal itself. All the options depend on great grilled vegetables.

Getting really good grilled vegetables that are tasty and cooked to perfection takes four important things:

1. Heat - lots of heat; your oven must be at 450 degrees, grill must be on high and grill pans must be heated on medium for five minutes before starting. You want enough heat to caramelize the natural sugars in the vegetables and to soften them but you don't want to over char or under cook them.

2. The right equipment - For indoor grilling I use something called a "scan pan" that works well, puts grill lines on the vegetables and does not require any added oil. A "Griddle Q" attachment will turn your outdoor grill into an almost commercial grill for vegetables and many other things. It will get extremely hot and will hold a lot of vegetables at one time. Google it online to check it out.

3. The right timing - For most vegetables it's usually more than three minutes. It's important to know what to watch for, when to turn them and it requires the development of a little bit of technique. Time and experience makes a difference. Your eye will become trained as to how they should look for your taste.

4. Cut to the right thickness or shape for your equipment; cut too thin and they will burn, cut too thick and they won't cook through. Thickness or thinness varies depending on the vegetable.

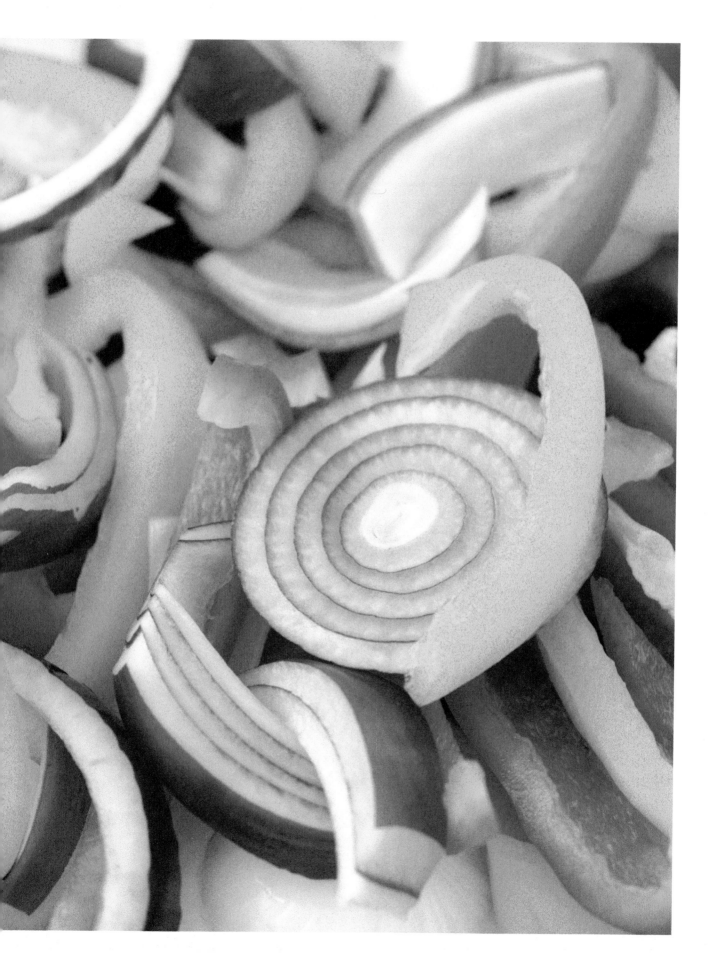

A small portion of my family's home near Naples in the small town of Nocelleto

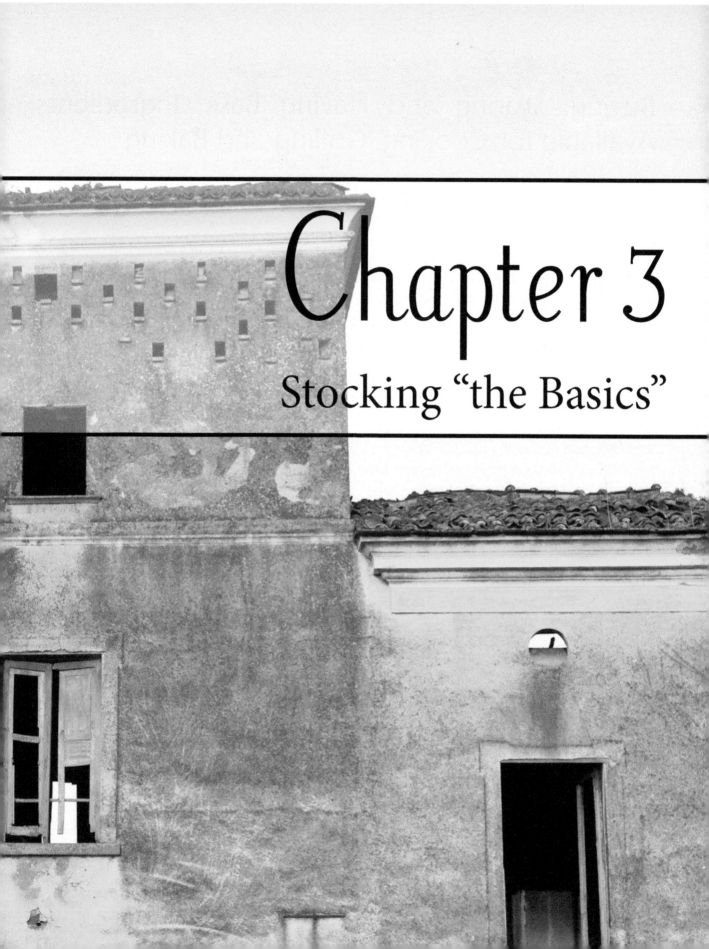

Chapter 3

Stocking "the Basics"

Buying, Storing and Having Basic Ingredients Available for Cooking, Grilling and Baking

Having your ingredients organized and keeping them fresh is the first step in gaining confidence and staying on track. There is nothing worse than coming home from work or any busy day, being hungry, and not having the ingredients and supplies to put together even the simplest meal.

Even worse is opening your cupboard only to find half opened bags and boxes of ingredients falling over on your cupboard shelves.

I recommend investing in glass storage jars. You can easily use canning jars of all sizes. I use a combination of canning and Bormioli jars. I like Bormioli jars because they come in various sizes with great caps that are easy to remove. The use of a large funnel is essential for transferring your grains, flours and baking essentials into the jars.

Store like ingredients together. Here I have my baking nuts, seeds, date sugar and raw cacao nibs in one place for use.

You'll want to keep the "basics" of nuts, grains and seeds on hand allowing for greater efficiency when making recipes. Here's a good "starter list" of ingredients that you will find in many of the recipes that follow.

Following is a recommended list of basic pantry items to keep on hand. It's not an exhaustive list of everything you will ever need but with these basics you will be able to put together a meal at any time.

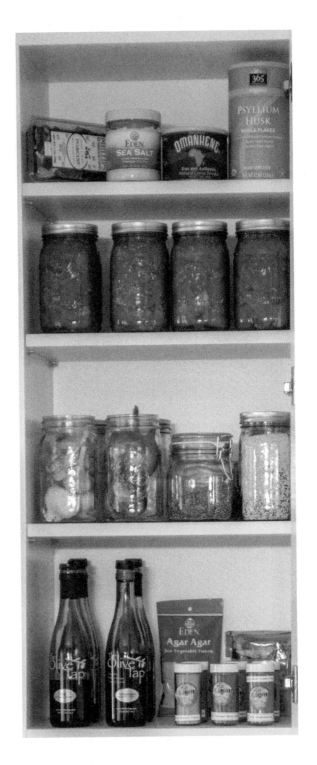

Whole Grains:

Rolled Oats – not quick oats

Short grain brown rice

Quinoa – red, brown or white

Beans and Legumes:

Garbanzo (chickpea)

Fava

Black beans

French lentils

Red, yellow and orange lentils

Nuts and Seeds:

Walnuts

Almonds

Pine nuts

Hazelnuts

Cashews

Pumpkin seeds

Sunflower seeds

Sesame seeds

Flax

Chia

Hemp Hearts

Note: All nuts as seeds should be raw

Dried Fruit:

Black raisins

Golden raisins

Mission Figs

Cranberries sweetened with apple juice

Cherries, unsweetened

Baking Supplies:

Unsweetened and if possible raw cocoa powder

Vanilla extract and/or vanilla paste

Whole vanilla bean

Date sugar

Baking soda without aluminum

Baking powder without aluminum

Apple cider vinegar

Maple syrup – grade B if possible

Cacao Nibs

Dried shredded coconut

Arrowroot

Fresh Produce:

Green onions

Arugula

Bok choy

Asparagus

Apple

Carrots

Celery

Avocado

Lemons

Bell peppers, red, yellow, orange

Onions – red and yellow

Fresh Garlic

Shallots

Flat parsley

Acorn Squash

Butternut Squash

Spinach

Kale

Swiss Chard

Watercress

Cauliflower

Sea Vegetables:

Kombu – simmer in stocks and soups – adds minerals also helps to digest beans

Nori – comes in pressed sheets or flakes for sprinkling over food or mixing with nuts

Non Dairy Milk: best if made at home

Almond

Oat

Rice

Cashew

Hemp

Spices and Herbs:

Dried oregano

Pepper corns

Thyme

Turmeric

Saffron

Black cumin

Cinnamon

Cloves

Red pepper flakes

Frozen:

Pineapple

Mango

Blueberries

Mixed Vegetables:

Peas

Corn

Green Beans

Miscellaneous:

Kalamata olives

Balsamic vinegar – aceto and fig are good starters

White balsamic vinegar

Hummus

Kitchen basics brand vegetable stock

Basic Spices for Flavor and Nutritional Value

A plant based diet need never taste bland and without a doubt recipes in this book will prove that point. Spices not only add flavor they also can also dazzle your taste buds. While spices make foods taste great it's easy to forget they can add a good dose of important antioxidants and phytochemicals to your foods.

Most people know herbs and spices add distinctive flavors often associated with particular cuisines. But little do people know that the red, yellow, and brown spices they sprinkle on their food - not to mention the herbs they cook with, also provide significant health benefits. After all, herbs and spices come from plants, and many plants, as scientists are discovering, contain a variety of healing substances, often found in high concentrations in their seeds, oils and other plant parts which make up herbs and spices.

For example, you may not consider basil, oregano or sage as "spices" because when they are fresh they are called "herbs." However, when they are dried they are considered spices. Remember drying herbs concentrates the flavor of the plant intensifying them as spices. It's unfortunate that the use of herbs for both their nutritional and taste value has been largely lost in the American diet. Experiment a little and you will be surprised at the exciting variations you can create.

The list below is not exhaustive but these should

be staples for their nutritional properties and their taste.

Black Cumin (formally known as Nigella sativa)

Studies show that black cumin may help prevent and treat a wide range of chronic illnesses, including cancer and heart disease. The star component of black cumin is a uniquely potent antioxidant called thymoquinone – a compound yet to be detected in any other plant. Black cumin seeds were found in King Tut's tomb. Many westernized countries are just rediscovering the powerful antioxidant properties of black cumin.

Cayenne

Contains capsaicin, which is the active ingredient in many prescriptions and over the counter creams, ointments and patches for arthritis and muscle pain. Over time, it short circuits pain by depleting nerve cells of a chemical called substance P which helps transmit pain signals along the nerve endings to the brain.

Cinnamon

One of the most powerful healing spices, cinnamon has become most famous for its ability to improve blood sugar control in people with diabetes. Some of its natural compounds improve insulin function, significantly lowering blood sugar with as little as ¼ to ½ teaspoons a day. Like many other spices, cinnamon has antibacterial and anti-inflammatory properties and is rich in antioxidants called polyphenols. Cinnamon also contains lots of fiber.

Cloves

Cloves contain the anti-inflammatory chemical called eugenol, which inhibits COX-2, a protein that spurs inflammation (the same protein that so-called COX-2 inhibitor drugs such as Celebrex quash). Cloves also rank high in antioxidants in one study. The combination of anti-inflammatory and antioxidant properties spells heaps of benefits, from boosting protection from heart disease to helping stave off cancer, as well as slowing the cartilage and bone damage caused by arthritis.

Coriander

Coriander seeds have been used for thousands of years as a digestive aid. The herb can be helpful for some people with irritable bowel syndrome, as it calms spasms that can lead to diarrhea. Preliminary test in animals supports traditional use for coriander as an anti-anxiety herb. Acts as an antioxidant, though you get the most punch from the leaf, cilantro.

Garlic

The famous odor of garlic comes from allycin, the sulfur compound believed to be responsible for most of the herbs medicinal benefits. When eaten daily, garlic can help lower heart disease risk by as much as 76 percent. How? By moderately reducing cholesterol levels (between 5 to 10 percent in some studies), by thinning the blood and thereby staving off dangerous clots and by acting as an antioxidant.

Garlic's sulfur compounds seem to ward off cancer, especially stomach and colorectal. Strong antibacterial and antifungal.

Ginger

Used for centuries in Asia as a digestive aid, researchers today are more excited about ginger's ability to combat inflammation. Several studies found that ginger (and turmeric) reduces pain and swelling in people with arthritis. It may work against migraines by blocking inflammatory substances called prostaglandins. Because it reduces inflammation, it may play a role in preventing and slowing the growth of cancer.

Mustard

Mustard comes from the seed of a plant in the cabbage family - a strong anticancer group of plants. Mustard seeds contain compounds that studies suggest may inhibit the growth of cancer cells. Mustard also packs enough heat to break up congestion. Like cayenne pepper, it has the ability to deplete nerve cells of substance P, a chemical that transmits pain signals to the brain when used externally.

Nutmeg

Like cloves, nutmeg contains eugenol, a compound that may benefit the heart. Medically nutmeg and mace have strong antibacterial properties. Myristicin, the active ingredient in nutmeg has hallucinatory effects if too much is ingested. The same active ingredient has been shown to inhibit an enzyme that contributes to Alzheimer's disease.

Sage

Known as a memory enhancer, sage in some studies has been shown to protect the brain against certain processes that lead to Alzheimer's disease.

Like so many other herbs, sage has strong anti-inflammatory, antioxidant as well as anticancer properties.

Saffron

Saffron has been reported to help lower cholesterol and keep cholesterol levels healthy. Animal studies have shown saffron to lower cholesterol by as much as 50%. Saffron has antioxidant properties; it is, therefore, helpful in maintaining healthy arteries and blood vessels. Saffron is also known to have anti-inflammatory properties, which are beneficial to cardiovascular health. The people of Mediterranean countries, where saffron use is common, have lower than normal incidence of heart diseases. From saffron's cholesterol lowering benefits to its anti-inflammatory properties, saffron may be one of the best supplements for cardiac health.

Turmeric

The spice that gives Indian curry its color, is used in Indian medicine. Lately, turmeric has been given attention as an anti-inflammatory and a strong cancer fighter. The chemical responsible for turmeric's golden color, called curcumin, is considered a top anticancer agent, helping to quell the inflammation that contributes to tumor growth. Lab studies show turmeric helps stop the growth and spread of cancer cells that do form. Studies have linked turmeric to reduced inflammation in a number of conditions, including, psoriasis. In animal studies, curcumin decreased the formation of amyloid, the stuff that makes up the brain deposits characteristic in people with Alzheimer's disease.

References:

http://herbalmusings.com/20-top-herbs-for-he...

Downregulation of tumor necrosis factor and other proinflammatory biomarkers by polyphenols: Subash C. Gupta, Amit K. Tyagi, Priya Deshmukh-taskar, Myriam Hinojosa, Bharat B. Aggarwal; Cytokine Research Laboratory, Department of Experimental Therapeutics, The University of Texas M.D. Anderson Cancer Center, Houston TX, 2014

Curcumin, a component of golden spice: From bedside to bench and back; Shade Prasad, Sub ash C. Gupta, Amit K. Tragi, Bharat B. Aggarwal, Biotechnology Advances 2014.

Bioavailability of herbs and spices in humans as determined by ex vivo inflammatory suppression and DNA strand breaks: Percival SS1, Vanned Heave JP, Nieves CJ, Montero C, Migliaccio AJ, Meadors J., Journal of Am Coll Nutrition, 2012.

Healing Spices, Bharat B. Aggarwal, PhD

Your shelves should look something like on page 14. Storing in glass jars keeps your ingredients fresher, organized and with one glance you'll be able to tell what needs replenishing.

The refrigerator is an extension of cupboards for fruits, vegetables and cooking basics. Avocados, beets, carrots, celery, herbs, lemons, limes, greens of all kinds and ginger to name a few. Be sure to use foods that may be at their peak for recipes and rotate for freshness.

The freezer is a great place to store items that would normally be kept in the pantry but are used less often. Nuts, whole grains, hemp seeds, raw cacao nibs are a few costly ingredients that you will want to avoid wasting. Also, in the summer months when the house may become a bit hotter using the freezer avoids rancidity.

While most people might consider the pantry as a place to store food items I use mine for storing equipment. The shelving I use is on wheels and when I'm doing a lot of cooking at one time I roll everything out of the "pantry" and right next to the kitchen counter and sink allowing easier access and quicker clean up.

The pantry looks like this:

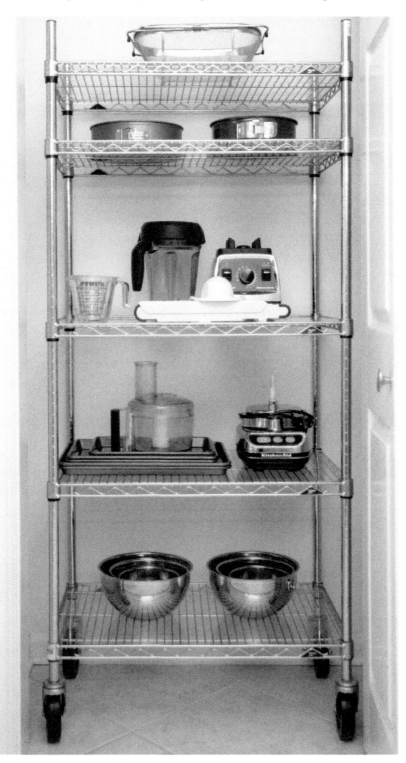

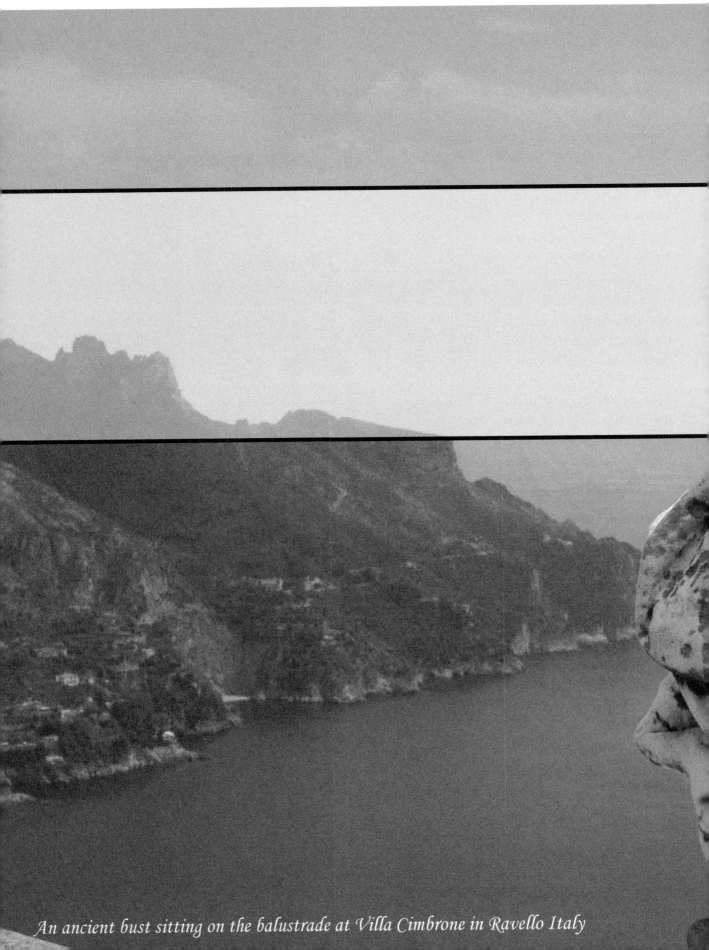

An ancient bust sitting on the balustrade at Villa Cimbrone in Ravello Italy

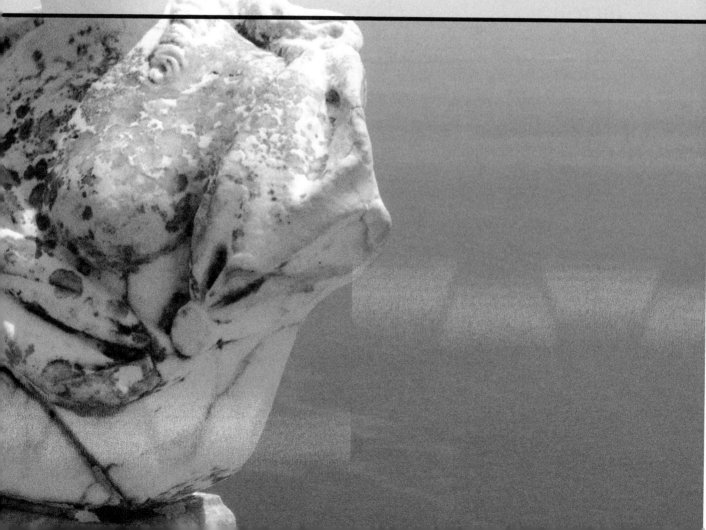

Chapter 4

Breakfast

Banana Oatmeal Muffins

These can be made ahead of time and will keep for two days. They make a lovely addition to breakfast or a simple breakfast themselves.

55 minutes prep time includes baking time
makes 12 small muffins or 6 large

Ingredients

- 3 cups of oatmeal (or oat bran)
- 1 teaspoon baking powder
- ¼ cup of maple syrup
- 1 granny smith apple, grated or chopped coarsely
- 4 very ripe bananas, chopped coarsely
- ¼ cup walnuts
- ¼ cup raisins or you can substitute dried cranberries for additional flavor
- ¾ cup water

Directions

1. Preheat oven to 350 degrees.
2. Mix the oatmeal (or oat bran) and baking powder in a large bowl.
3. Add all remaining ingredients to the oatmeal except for the water. Add the water last making sure the batter is not too wet or too dry. You may need to reserve some out or add more.
4. Bake in cupcake tins for a smaller size or large parchment cups for larger muffins. Bake large muffins for about 45 minutes and smaller size muffins for 35 minutes, or until you see that the tops are brown and middle is firm.

Tip: Be sure to find a baking powder that does not contain aluminum.

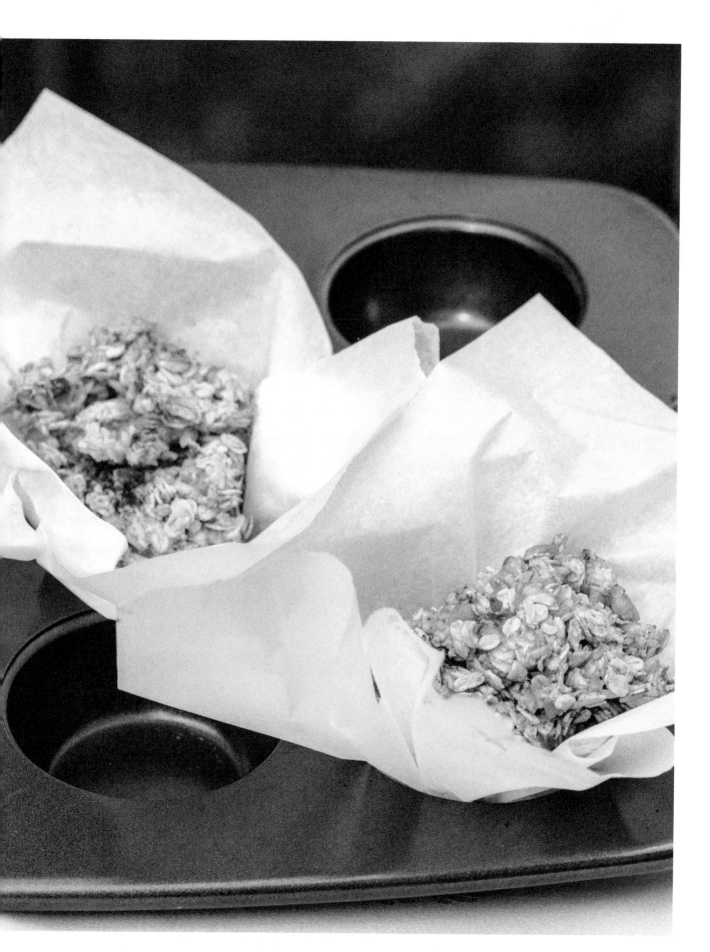

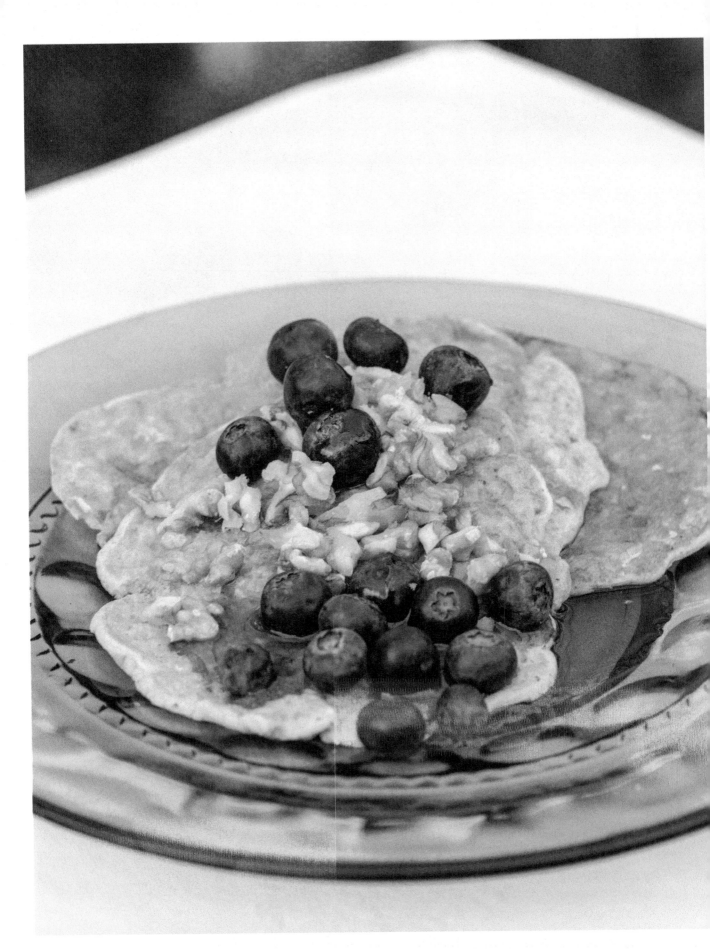

Oat and Garbanzo Bean Flour Pancakes

These are lovely and usually reserved for Sunday morning at my house. You can add a variety of toppings to make them as simple or complex as you would like. I've used various fruit spreads for toppings, a mixture of raspberries, blueberries and strawberries and sometimes just coarsely chopped walnuts. The maple syrup in the photo is grade B. These are naturally gluten free.

25 minutes prep time
makes about 8 pancakes

Ingredients

- ½ cup oat flour (see second step)
- ½ cup garbanzo bean flour
- 1 tablespoon baking powder
- 1 teaspoon maple sugar
- 2 tablespoons ground flax
- 3 tablespoons water
- 1 ½ cups oat milk
- Real maple syrup or fruit for topping (optional)

Directions

1. Mix the ground flax and water together in a small bowl and let the mixture sit for 5 minutes.
2. Make your oat flour by processing ½ cup of oats in your food processor for about 30 seconds. The "flour" will have some texture to it and that's OK.
3. Combine the dry ingredients in a bowl and whisk together.
4. In a separate bowl stir together the flax and water mixture with the oat milk.
5. Add the liquid to the dry ingredients and stir well.
6. Preheat a nonstick skillet (not a coated skillet but one that is made of material that is nonstick).
7. Once the skillet is hot, place a scant ¼ cup of batter into the skillet and cook until you see bubbles forming on top. Turn the pancake over and cook until browned on both sides.
8. Top with your preferred topping or even a sparse amount of real maple syrup.

Tip: If you can't find maple sugar then date sugar makes a great substitute.

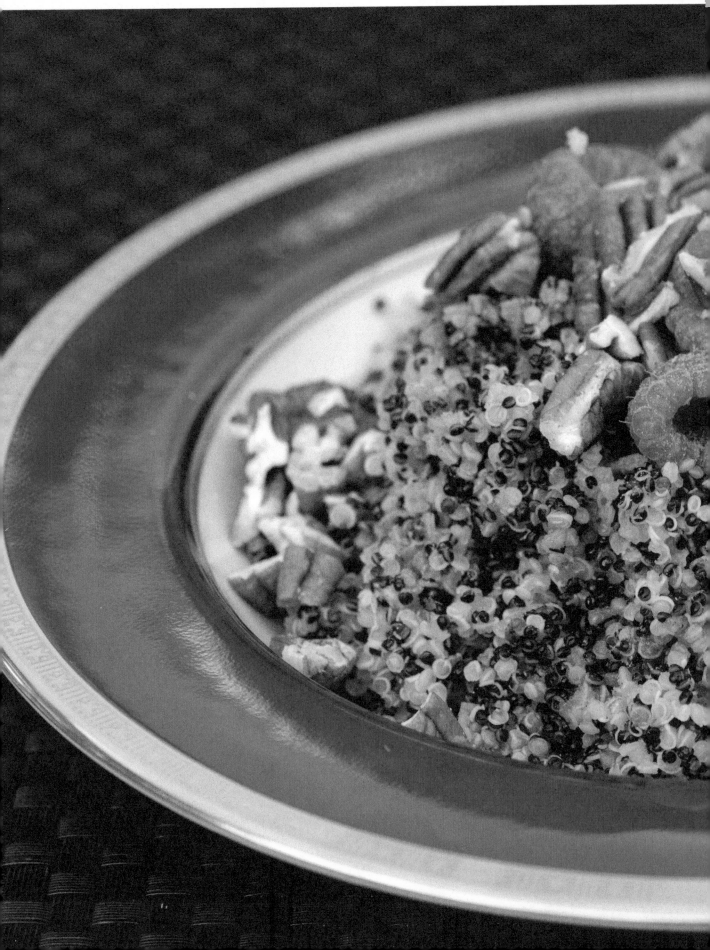

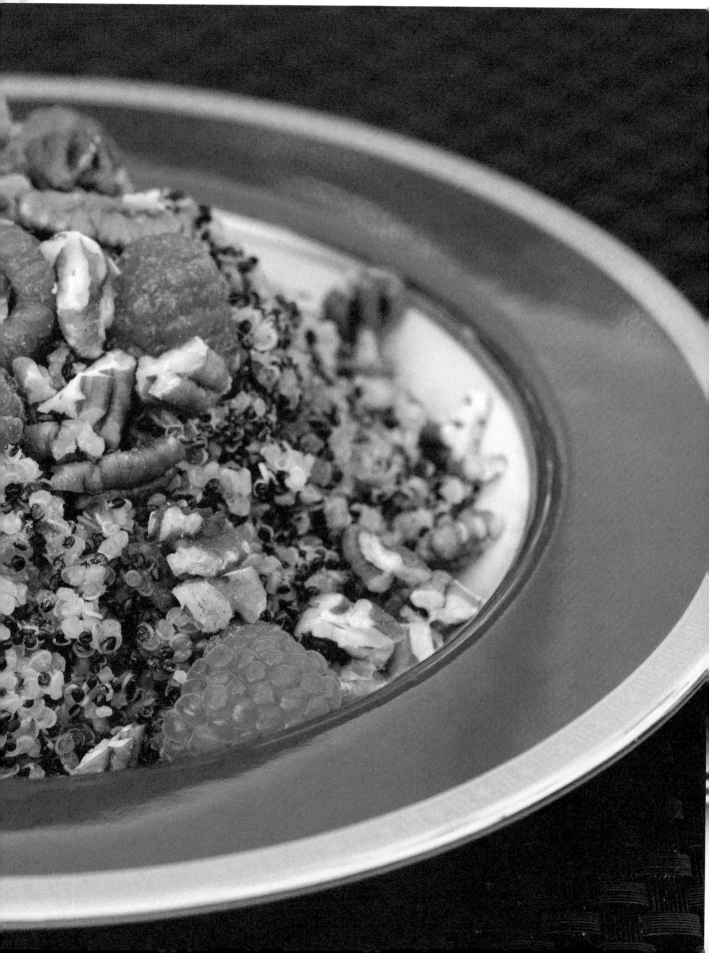

Warm Quinoa, Berry and Cinnamon Breakfast

A lovely light but satisfying high protein breakfast. You can substitute other berries for the blueberries or combine additional ones such as raspberries and blackberries.

about 20 minutes prep time
makes 4 servings

Ingredients

- 1 cup non-dairy milk
- 1 cup water
- 1 cup quinoa, rinsed using a fine strainer before using
- 2 cups fresh blueberries
- ½ teaspoon ground cinnamon, freshly ground if possible
- ⅓ cup lightly toasted pecans or walnuts, toast for 5-6 minutes in a dry skillet)
- 1 tablespoon maple syrup or fruit (optional for topping)

Directions

1. Combine the water and non-dairy milk in a medium saucepan. Add the quinoa and bring to a boil. Reduce the heat to low-medium and simmer about 15 minutes. The liquid should be absorbed and the quinoa moist. Quinoa gets very dry when over cooked.
2. Cover the saucepan and let stand for 5 minutes.
3. Stir in the blueberries, toasted nuts and cinnamon.
4. Separate into 4 bowls and top with a drizzle of maple syrup if desired.

No Cook Make Ahead Breakfast

This is quick and easy to put together in the evening and is lovely to have in the morning.

5 minutes prep time
makes 1 generous serving

Ingredients

- 1 cup uncooked old fashioned oatmeal
- 1 cup almond milk
- 2 tablespoons chopped walnuts or almonds
- 2 tablespoons ground flaxseed
- 2 tablespoons sesame seeds
- 8 ounces fresh berries
- 1 apple coarsely chopped

Directions

1. In a large bowl mix together the dry ingredients with the milk. Cover and place in the refrigerator overnight.
2. In the morning, add the berries and chopped apple.

Chia Breakfast Pudding

This is a tasty and filling breakfast with many options for variety. The recipe is kept simple with blueberry and walnut toppings but other berries and banana can be used as well, let your imagination go. As you can see you can make it as elegant as you would like by serving it in a fancy glass.

5 minutes prep time
makes 2 generous servings

Ingredients

- 1 ½ cup almond milk
- ¼ cup chia seeds
- Fruits for topping (optional)

Directions

1. Mix the almond milk with the chia seeds and let the mixture sit for about 10 minutes.
2. Spoon into serving dishes and top with fruit as desired.
3. You can make this recipe the night before and refrigerate overnight. Use less chia seeds if making ahead as it will become thicker the longer it sits.

Tip: It's preferable to use homemade almond milk but other commercial non-dairy milk is also acceptable. You can also adjust the amount of chia seeds to make the pudding thicker by adding more chia seeds or thinner by using less.

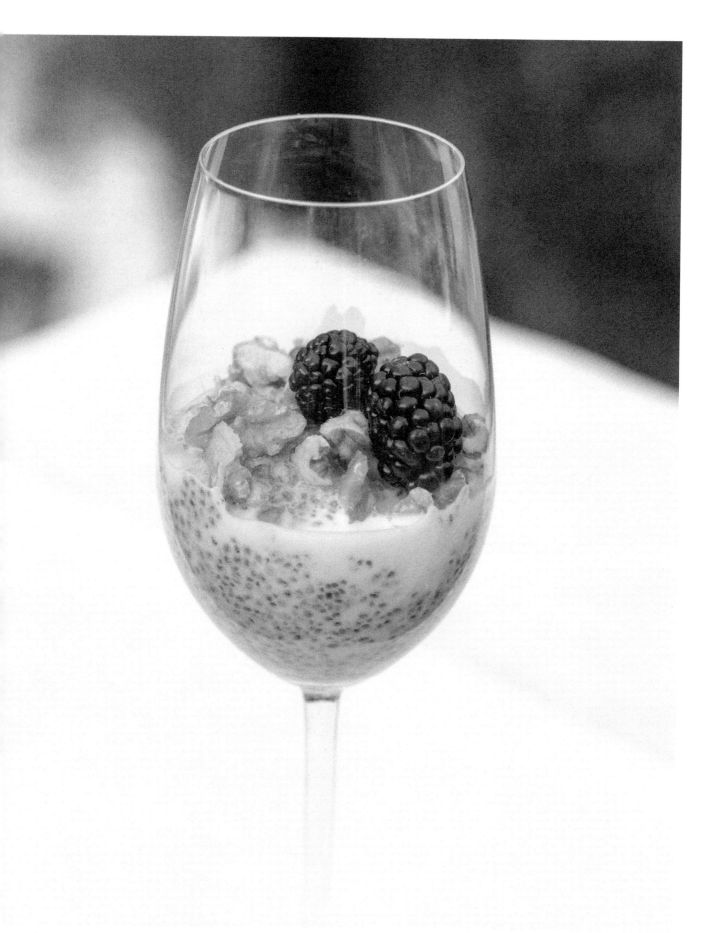

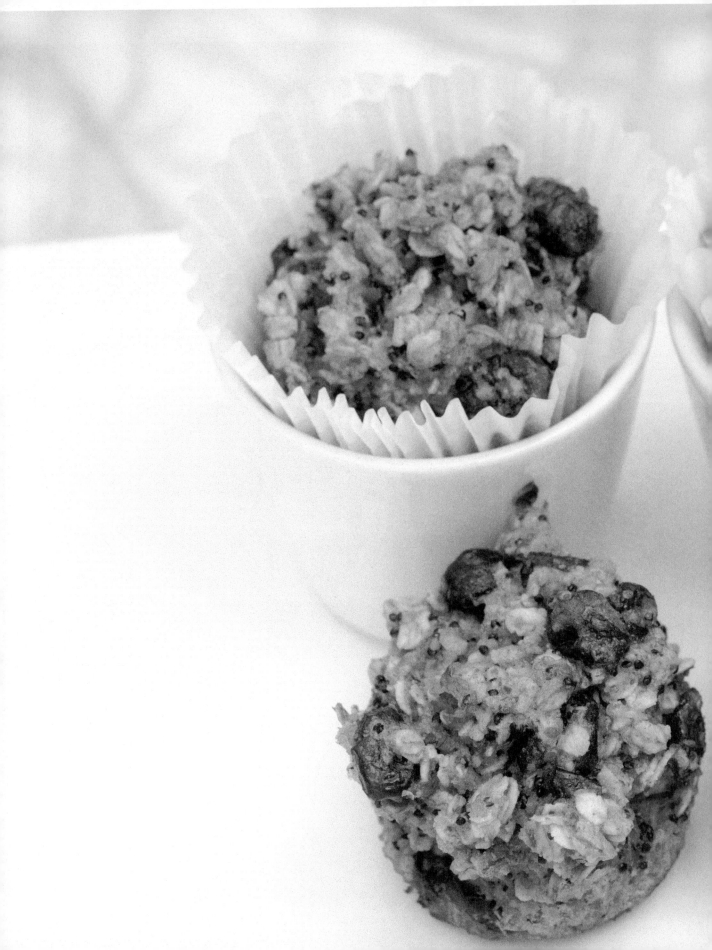

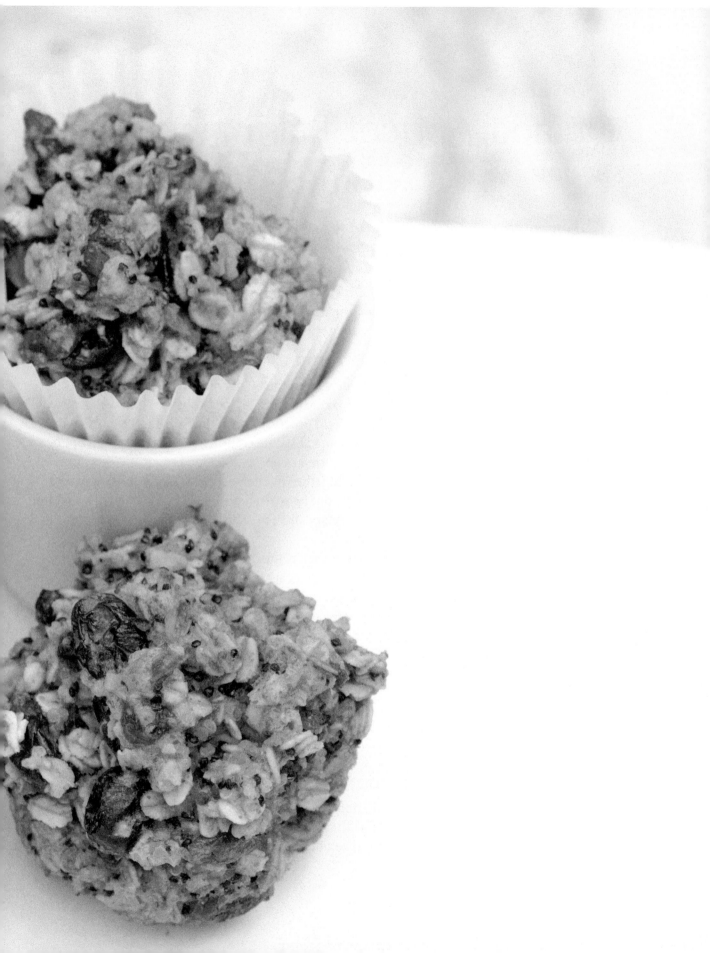

Quinoa-Apricot Raisin and Nut Muffins

These are great as a snack in a small size or as a great breakfast muffin as shown. If you prefer a sweeter muffin and one that is less crunchy, add ½ cup of unsweetened apple sauce to the batter.

about 20 minutes prep time if using apricot spread instead of making apricot paste

makes 2 dozen small muffins or 8-10 large

Ingredients

- ½ cup apricot paste
- ¾ cup cooked quinoa
- 1 ½ cups oatmeal
- ½ cup ground nuts (I used pecans but walnuts are even more nutritious and you can blend nuts with sunflower seeds if preferred)
- ½ cup golden raisins
- ¼ cup almond butter
- 2 tablespoons ground flaxseed
- 4 tablespoons warm water
- ½ cup almond milk (see page 164)
- ¼ teaspoon cinnamon
- 2 teaspoons pure vanilla extract

Directions

1. Preheat oven to 350 degrees.
2. To make your apricot paste blend ½ cup dried apricots in a food processor until they are a paste consistency. You can substitute commercial apricot spread but be sure to find one without added sugar.
3. Mix together the flaxseed with warm water and set aside, but be sure to stir it every so often while making this recipe. It should be gooey like the consistency of an egg.
4. The quinoa is finished when there is no water left in the pan, once it reaches this stage stir together the cooked quinoa, oats, nuts and raisins.
5. Process together in a food processor the almond butter, apricot paste, flaxseed meal, almond milk, cinnamon and vanilla
6. Fold this mixture in with the dry ingredients and stir well. Batter should be firm to the touch.
7. Bake for 18 minutes or until golden brown on top and cooked through.

Tip: You can always substitute dried cranberries for the golden raisins but keep in mind dried cranberries almost always have added sugar whereas the raisins do not. If you do use dried cranberries try to find ones that are sweetened with apple juice and not sugar. You can usually find them in the bulk aisle of the grocery store or at Whole Foods or similar stores.

High Fiber Chia Breakfast Pudding

This version of chia pudding has additional benefits of more omega-3 fatty acids from the flax seed, more fiber from the pepita seeds and an additional pop of flavor from the raisins.

5 minutes prep time
makes 2 servings

Ingredients

- 1 cup almond milk (see page 164)
- 2 tablespoons of ground flax
- 2 tablespoons of chia seeds
- Raw pepita seeds to taste
- Raisins to taste

Directions

1. Grind whole flax seeds in food processor if not already ground. It is a good idea to buy flax seed whole and grind as needed in order to keep your ingredients fresher.
2. Soak the chia seeds in water for a few minutes. The longer you soak them the more they expand making them not only easier to digest but also creates a pudding like consistency depending on the amount of liquid that is added.

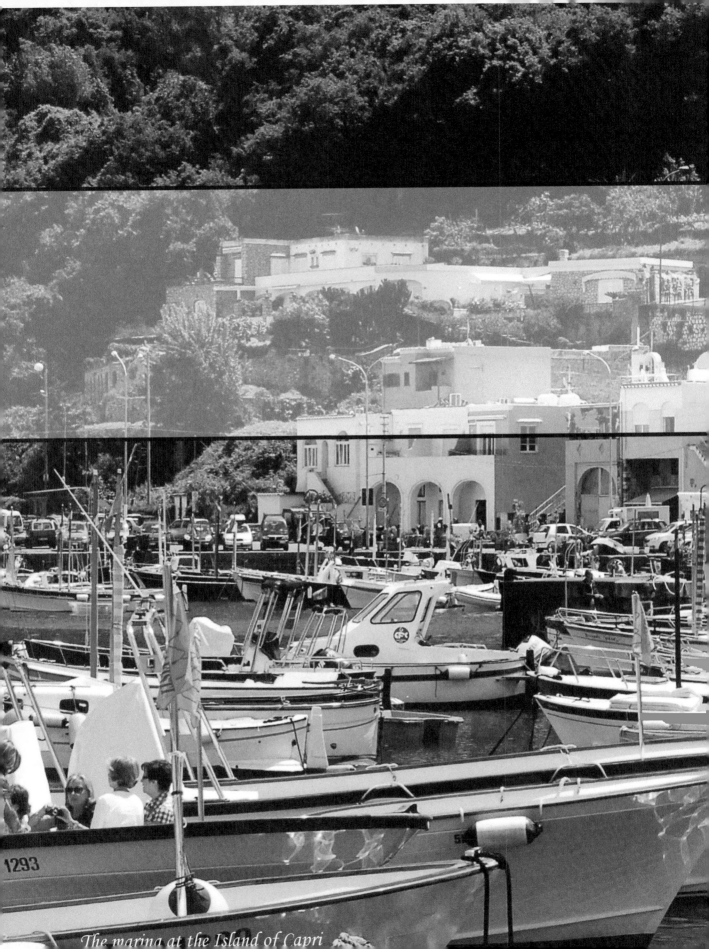

The marina at the Island of Capri

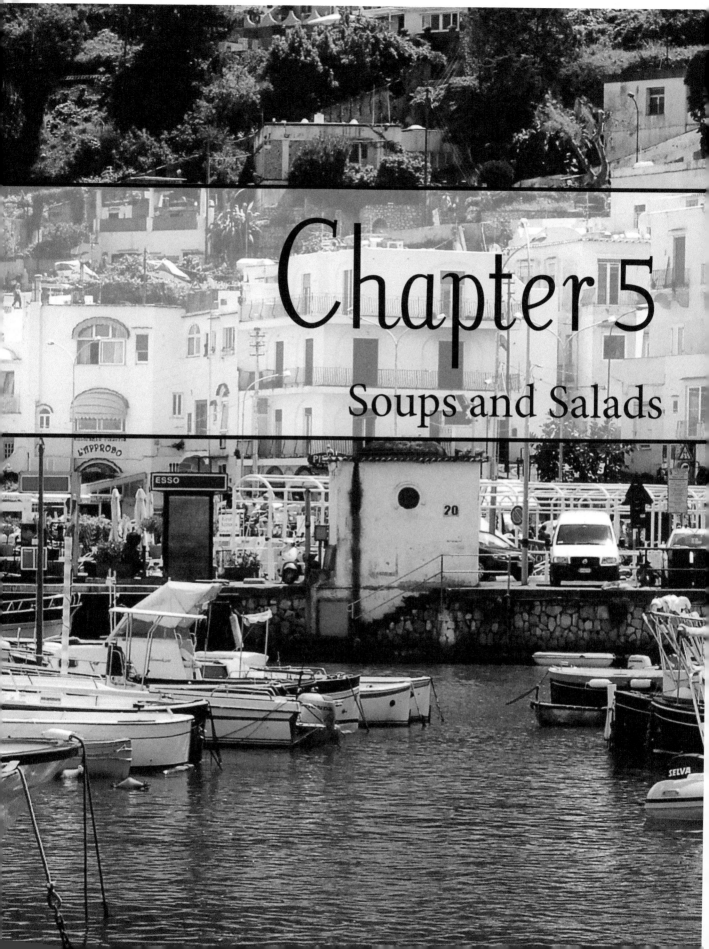

Chapter 5

Soups and Salads

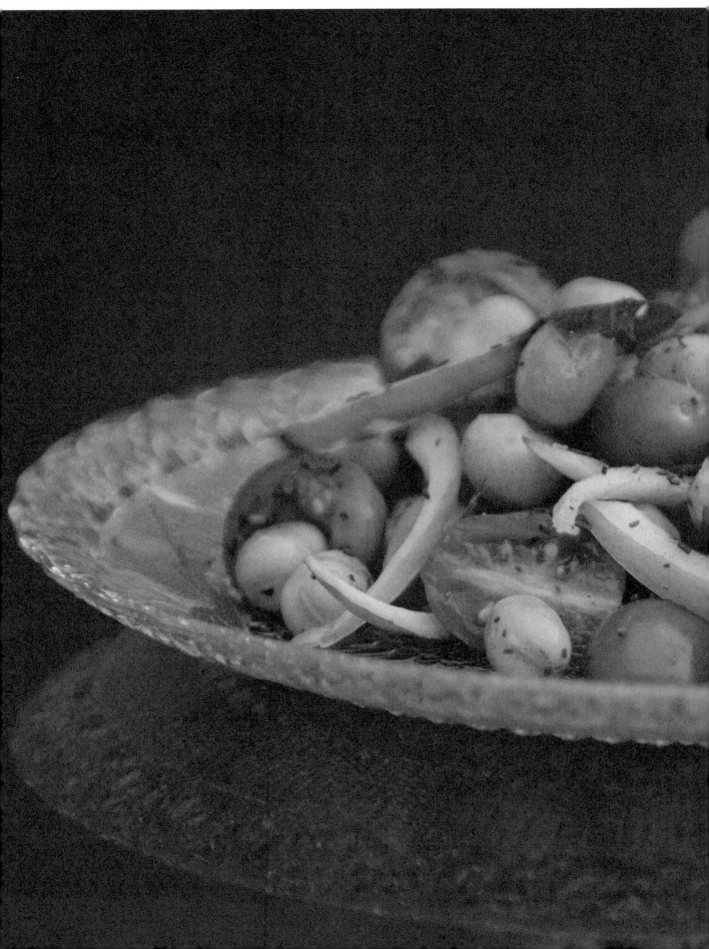

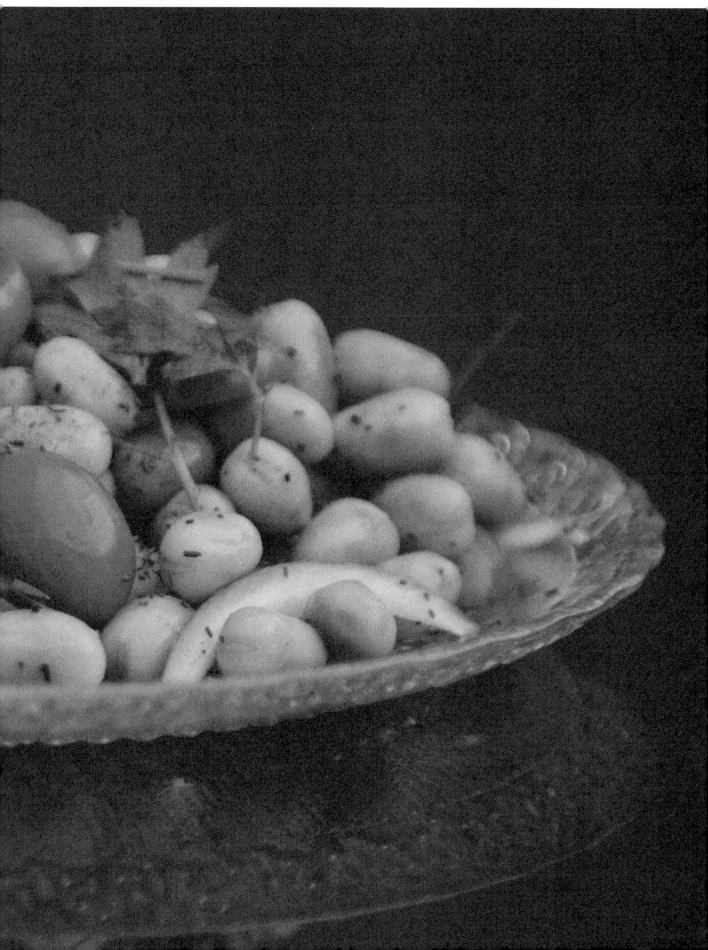

Fava Bean Salad

Fava beans add fiber, protein and other great nutrients. Beans are a staple of the longest living people on the globe. The addition of powerful antioxidants in black cumin makes this recipe which is already a nutritional powerhouse even better. It's so easy to make yet so beautiful to serve.

10 minutes prep time
makes 2 servings

Ingredients

- 1 cup fava beans
- ½ sweet onion, sliced thinly
- 1 cup cherry tomatoes, cut in half
- Juice from one lemon
- 2 tablespoons of good quality white balsamic vinegar
- 1 teaspoon ground black cumin
- Small handful of fresh parsley, chopped
- Sea salt and fresh ground pepper

Directions

1. Combine all ingredients (except for the lemon juice and vinegar) in a small bowl.
2. Toss together and add the lemon juice and balsamic vinegar on top.

Strawberry Bok Choy Salad

I love making dishes that present so elegantly as this one and yet are powerfully healthful. Quinoa delivers protein, walnuts add omega 3 and bok choy adds the powerful antioxidants of the cruciferous vegetable.

25 minutes prep time
makes 2 servings

Ingredients

- 3 tablespoons balsamic Vinegar. Use good quality vinegar – aceto balsamic works well, or for a creative touch, try this recipe with sour apple or Sicilian lemon balsamic vinegar. A lighter color balsamic (sour apple or lemon) pops the color of this dish as well.
- 1 teaspoon mustard
- 1 teaspoon good quality maple syrup
- 1 tablespoon shallot, finely chopped
- Salt and/or pepper to taste
- ¾ cup cooked quinoa, warmed
- ⅔ cup fresh strawberries, chopped in quarters
- 1½-2 cups bok choy, roughly chopped
- 2 tablespoons walnuts, lightly toasted and chopped

Directions

1. To make the dressing combine the vinegar, mustard, maple syrup, shallot and salt and/or pepper in a small bowl and mix well with a fork or whisk. You can also prepare this in a small jar and shake well to mix. For a more tart finish add more vinegar and for a sweeter finish add more maple syrup. Experiment with it to your liking.
2. Rinse the quinoa in a fine mesh colander. Cover with twice the amount of water (this is always the case when making quinoa) in a saucepan and bring to a boil. Stir once and reduce heat to a simmer. Cover and steam for about 15 minutes or until the water is absorbed. Remove from heat and fluff with a fork.
3. Place the bok choy at the bottom of a medium size bowl. Transfer the warm quinoa and place on top of the bok choy. This process slightly wilts the greens but keeps it crisp enough to taste fresh.
4. Add the strawberries (you can also use blueberries or other fruit in season) top with dressing and sprinkle walnuts on top.

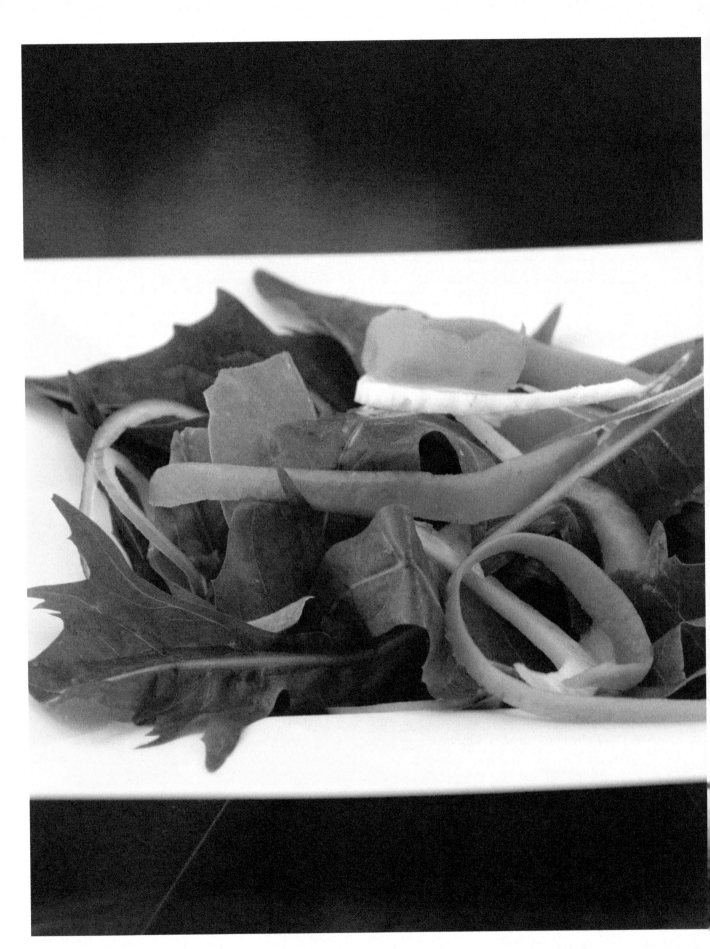

Arugula Salad with Fennel and Carrot Ribbons

This is a great simple salad recipe that can be assembled in minutes. You can easily add chickpeas and/or sunflower seeds to create a hearty side dish or light lunch.

10 minutes prep time
makes 2 generous servings

Ingredients

- 10 ounces baby arugula, baby spinach or similar green leafy vegetable
- 1 large fennel bulb, cored and sliced thinly
- 3 large carrots, peeled
- ½ red onion sliced thinly
- White balsamic vinegar to taste

Directions

1. Add arugula (or spinach) and fennel slices to a large bowl
2. Use a vegetable peeler and apply pressure to carrots creating "ribbons"
3. Add the carrots and red onion to the greens and fennel
4. Top with flavorful white balsamic vinegar – I use Sicilian Lemon balsamic vinegar

Apricot Almond Salad

Apricots and almonds are a great combination and the addition of lemony spicy ginger, the crunch of celery and the colorful pepper and onion is a beautiful example of eating a rainbow of colors for nutritional balance.

10 minutes prep time
makes 2 servings

Ingredients

- 1 clove garlic, minced
- 1 cup fresh apricots, (organically grown if possible)
- 1 red onion, diced
- 1 yellow pepper, diced
- 2 ribs of celery, diced
- 1T fresh basil
- 1 teaspoon fresh shredded ginger
- ⅓ cup slivered almonds, light-ly toasted
- Romaine lettuce leaves for serving

Directions

1. Combine all ingredients except the lettuce in a small bowl and toss together.
2. Prepare individual servings on a bed of crisp lettuce leaves

Tip: If you can't find fresh apricots then dried (unsulphured) will make a great substitute, just soak them for about 20 minutes to rehydrate them.

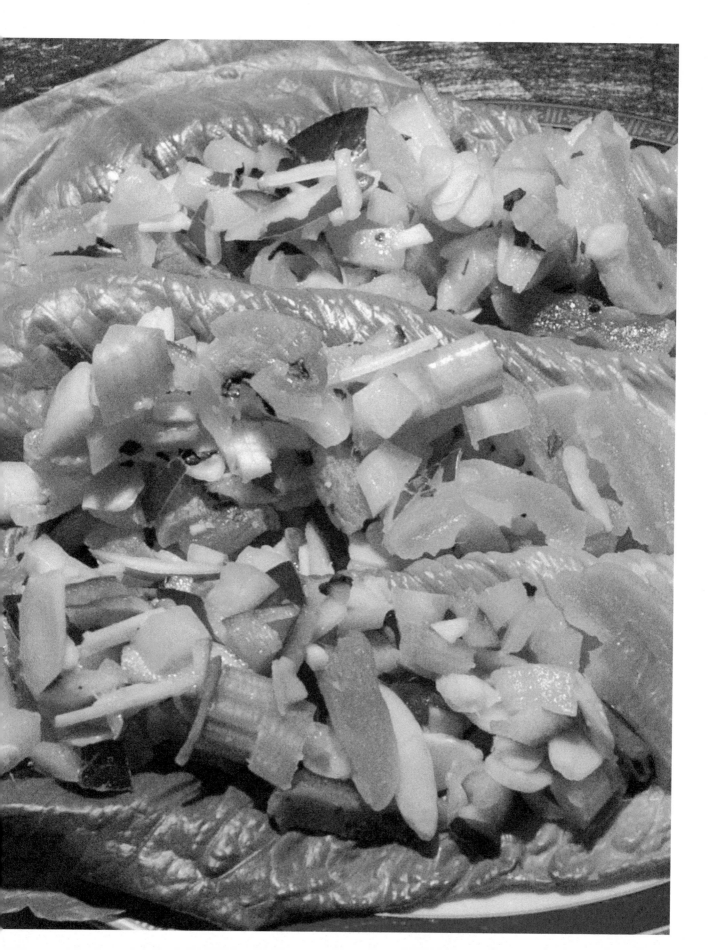

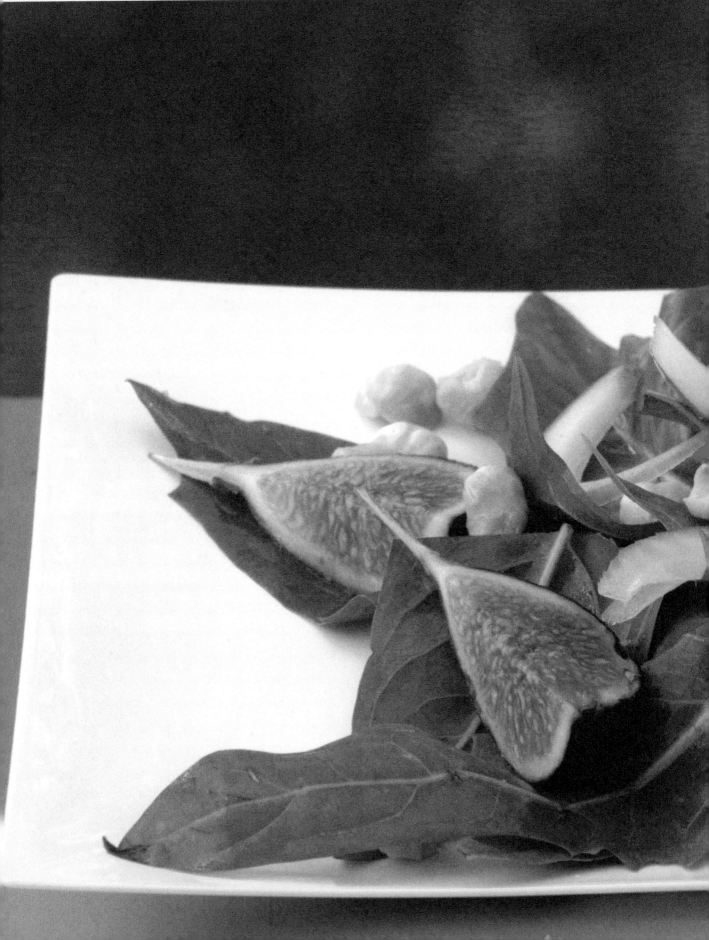

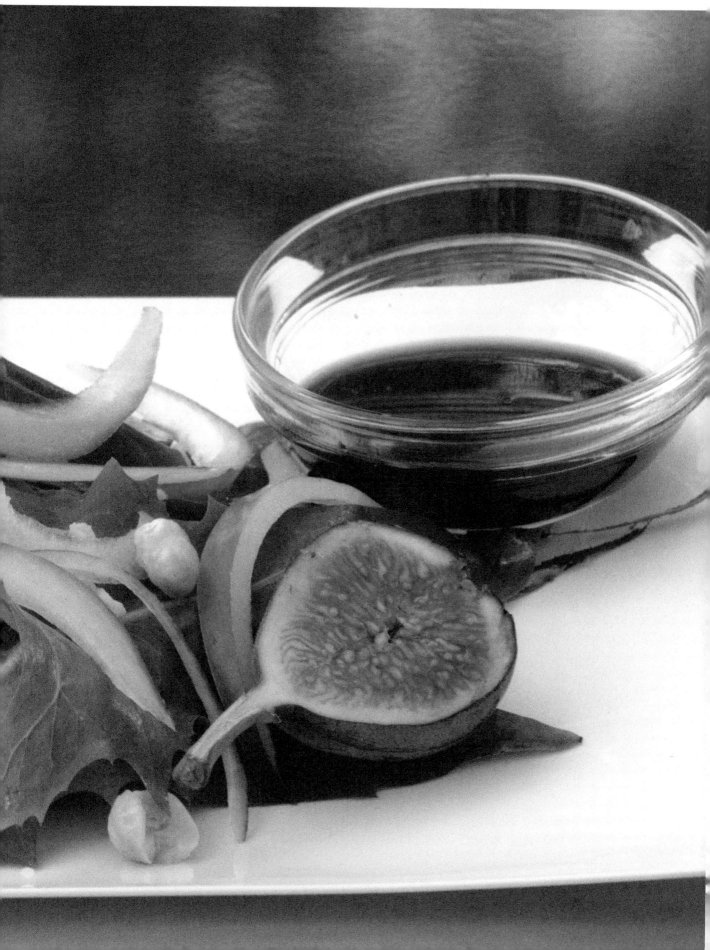

Elegant Fig Salad

Fresh figs are not always available but when you can find them this is a great way to enjoy them. I love serving this salad for dinner parties because it's always such a welcomed surprise from the ordinary.

20 minutes prep time
makes 4 servings

Ingredients

- 2 small red onions or shallots, (I prefer shallots) sliced in wide strips
- ¼ cup roasted hazelnuts (walnuts or almonds also work well)
- Large bunch of lettuce, (can be romaine or other salad greens) leaves torn roughly
- 2 cups of watercress or Arugula
- 6 ripe fresh figs
- Balsamic vinegar to taste
- Fresh ground black pepper to taste

Directions

1. Preheat the oven to 400 degrees. Line two roasting pans with parchment paper.
2. Slice the onions or shallots into wide strips and put them on one roasting tray and the hazelnuts on the other. Roast for 20 minutes turning the nuts and onions once or twice as needed to roast evenly. Remove pans from the oven and allow to cool. Break the roasted hazelnuts with the side of a big knife (This is easier than trying to slice them in half).
3. Assemble the salad on four individual plates. Mix the three salad leaves together and place a few on each plate. Cut the figs lengthways into four or six pieces and place a few fig pieces on each plate. Add some roasted onions or shallots on the leaves then top with more leaves and finally the remaining fig and onions or shallots. You want to build up the salad into a small pyramid.
4. Drizzle balsamic vinegar over the salad and finish with a scattering of toasted hazelnuts. Elegant, delicious and healthy!

Tip: Fig balsamic vinegar is heavenly with this recipe and has even become easier to find in stores.

Roasted Butternut Squash Soup

An easy-to-make soup that is loaded with nutrients and great taste!

1 hour prep time
makes 4 servings

Ingredients

- 4 cups butternut squash, cut in cubes
- 3 cups vegetable broth (I like Kitchen Basics Brand of broth, it has less sodium.)
- ¼ cups non-dairy milk (I use oat milk)
- 1-2 shallots, sautéed until transparent and soft
- Dash of red pepper flakes
- Freshly ground black pepper
- Pepita or pumpkin seeds for garnish

Directions

1. Preheat oven to 425 degrees and line a heavy (preferable metal) baking pan with parchment paper.
2. Spread squash in single layer in the pan. Use two baking pans lined with parchment if needed.
3. Roast for about 40 minutes or until tender when pierced with a fork. If you prefer you can also roast a whole butternut squash with the skin on in the oven for about 45 minutes or until skin is soft. It will be easy to peel, cut and will be ready for the food processor.
4. Transfer the roasted squash to a food processor, Vita Mix or heavy-duty blender. Add remaining ingredients and process until smooth.
5. If soup is too thick, add additional broth to reach desired consistency.
6. Divide among 4 bowls and garnish with roasted pepita seeds on top for additional texture and "crunch."

Tip: A variation of this soup can be made by substituting steamed asparagus for the squash and using less vegetable broth.

Roasted Pumpkin Soup

If you've never roasted a whole pumpkin in the oven it's easy and I highly recommend it. There's nothing like the smell of fresh roasted pumpkin in the house on a cool fall or winter day. You can place the pumpkin directly on the oven rack for roasting. You should turn it half way through baking so it roasts evenly.

50 minutes prep time, mostly roasting time for the pumpkin
makes 4 servings

Ingredients

- 1 small to medium sized pumpkin, enough to make 2 cups of pumpkin
- 3 leeks, chopped
- Salt and fresh ground pepper to taste
- 1 ¼ cup vegetable stock (Kitchen Basics is the best brand I've found that has the lowest salt content)
- ½ cup oat milk
- Cayenne pepper to taste
- Raw or toasted pepita seeds for topping

Directions

1. Preheat the oven to 400 degrees.
2. Set the whole pumpkin on the rack and roast for 45-50 minutes or until soft to the touch.
3. While the pumpkin is roasting slowly sauté the white part of the leeks over low to medium heat until browned and soft.
4. When the pumpkin is finished roasting, cut it open and remove the pumpkin flesh from the inside. Separate out the seeds.
5. Place the pumpkin flesh in a high speed food processor or a Vita Mix. Add the vegetable stock, leeks, oat milk and spices and blend at full speed to get the consistency of a smooth soup.
6. Divide into 4 bowls
7. Serve immediately or reheat when ready to serve and top with the pepitas or sunflower seeds.

Tip: You can keep the pumpkin seeds for a snack or as a topping by baking them separately in a 400 degree oven and if you prefer add a pinch of salt.

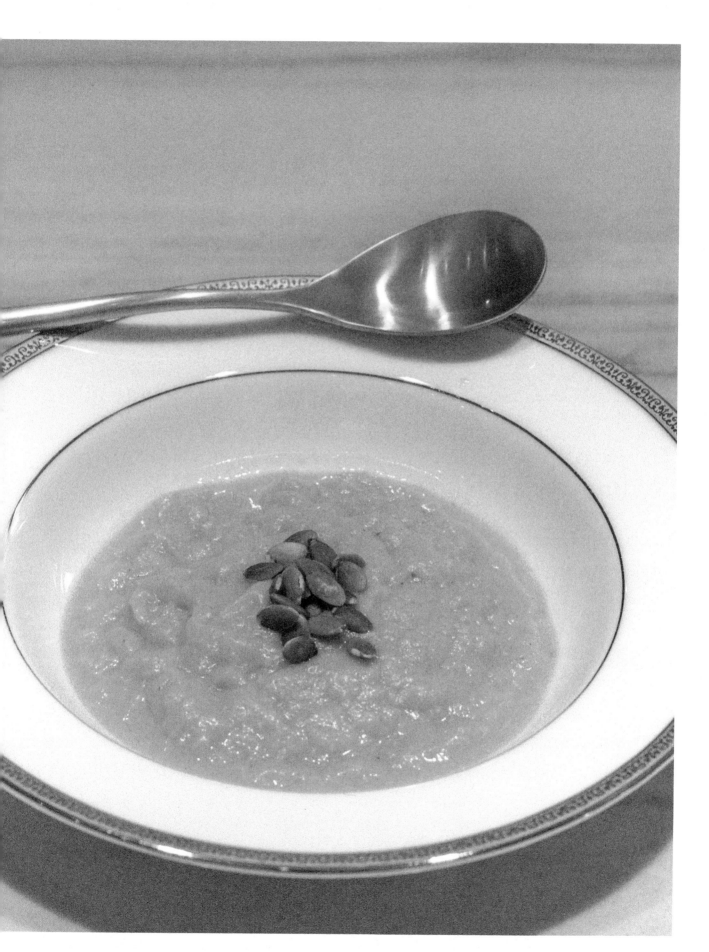

Cream of Asparagus Soup

A lovely creamy soup that is especially nice in the spring when asparagus is in season. Guests love it and I serve it as a first course at dinner parties.

30 minutes prep time
makes about 4 "appetizer" servings

Ingredients

- 1½ pounds of asparagus spears, lightly steamed
- 2 shallots or leeks, lightly sautéed until tender
- ½ cup non-dairy milk (I prefer cashew or oat milk)
- 1½ cup vegetable stock
- Salt and pepper to taste

Directions

1. Place all ingredients in a food processor or a Vita Mix, but reserve ½ cup of the asparagus tips for a garnish. Blend until smooth. If using a Vita Mix you may notice the soup gets a bit of air in it that causes it to "puff" up. You may need to stir it down a bit.
2. You may want to add additional vegetable stock and non-dairy milk until you have the desired consistency.
3. Serve in individual bowls and top with a few tips for garnish.

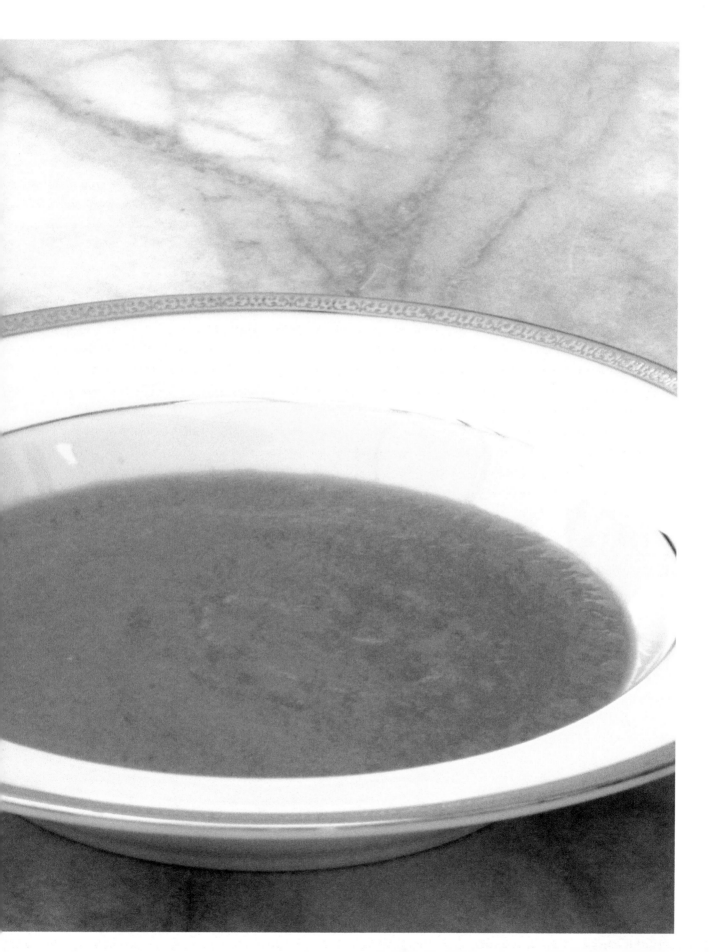

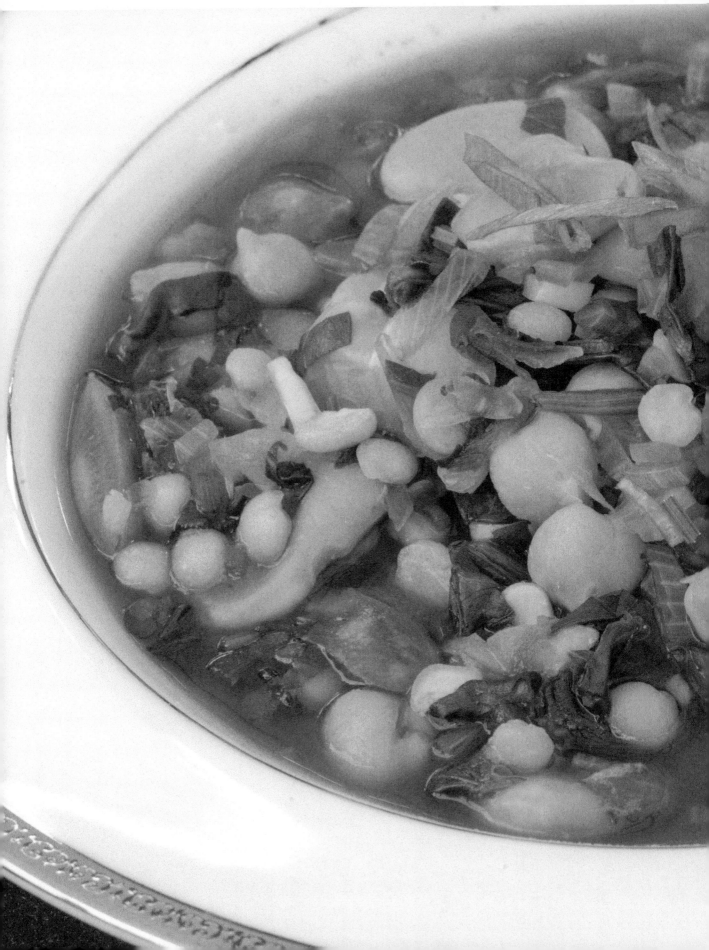

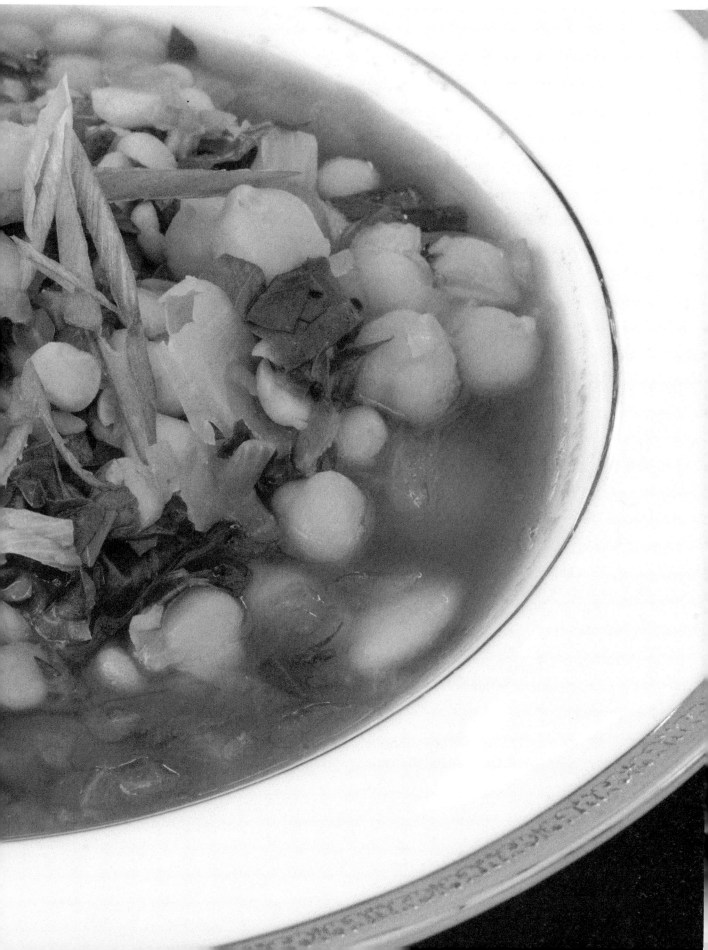

Rustic Bean and Lentil Soup

A hearty soup for a winter's evening or served in small portions as a first course for dinner. This soup crosses cultures between Italian and Middle Eastern cuisine and its rich and complex flavors are delightful!

1 hour prep time with prepared beans or overnight with dried beans

makes 4 servings

Ingredients

- 1 can chickpeas
- 1 cup lima beans, also called butter beans
- 1 cup yellow split peas, rinsed
- 2 large onions, sliced thinly
- 5-10 large cloves of garlic, sliced thinly
- 8 cups vegetable stock
- 1 cup flat leaf parsley, chopped roughly
- 6 green onions, sliced thin-ly using both the white and green parts
- 6 or 7 large handfuls of baby spinach leaves
- Salt and fresh ground black pepper to taste

Directions

1. Drain the beans and set aside.
2. Simmer the onion and garlic in a very large non stick pan until onions are translucent and garlic is softened. If preferred you can sauté the onions and garlic with ½ tablespoon oil.
3. Add the chickpeas and lima beans to the pan, then add the split peas and vegetable stock. Simmer for about 30 minutes. If a froth develops from the beans while simmering skim it off occasionally.
4. After 30 minutes add the parsley, green onions and spinach and simmer another 10 minutes. If the soup becomes too thick (which can happen if the beans become creamy) add more vegetable stock while doing the last simmering.
5. Add a pinch of salt and fresh ground pepper to taste. Enjoy!

Tip: When choosing your vegetable stock use homemade or Kitchen Basics brand. If neither are available find a good brand with the lowest amount of sodium.

Broccoli Leek Soup

This is a wonderful addition to a winter meal or a stand-alone dish for lunch. For additional texture and a bit of crunch, top with pumpkin or pepita seeds or serve with a healthy cracker. I use "Mary's Gone Crackers" brand.

20 minutes prep time (if using a prepared soup stock)
15 minutes cook time
makes 4 servings

Ingredients

- 2 leeks, finely chopped with some of the tender green portion as well
- 1½ pounds of broccoli, separate the florets and cut into pieces
- 4 cups of vegetable stock
- Pinch of salt and fresh ground pepper to taste

Directions

1. Warm the vegetable stock in a large pan.
2. Sauté the leeks in a non-stick pan for 3-5 minutes or until softened. Remove the leeks and sauté the broccoli. You may have to do this in two or three parts if your pan is small. Sauté the broccoli until lightly softened but still has good green color.
3. Add the leeks and broccoli to the vegetable stock and bring to a simmer. Cook until vegetables are tender.
4. When the vegetables are tender puree the soup in batches using a Vita Mix, blender or a stick blender.
5. Once it is pureed, reheat the soup gently, season with salt and white pepper and ladle into warm bowls.

Tip: You can prepare your own with water and simmering whatever vegetables you have or you can purchase a good vegetable stock. The brand I use is Kitchen Basics. It has the lowest salt content of any prepared stock. If you can use fresh white pepper to grind it's nicer for the presentation.

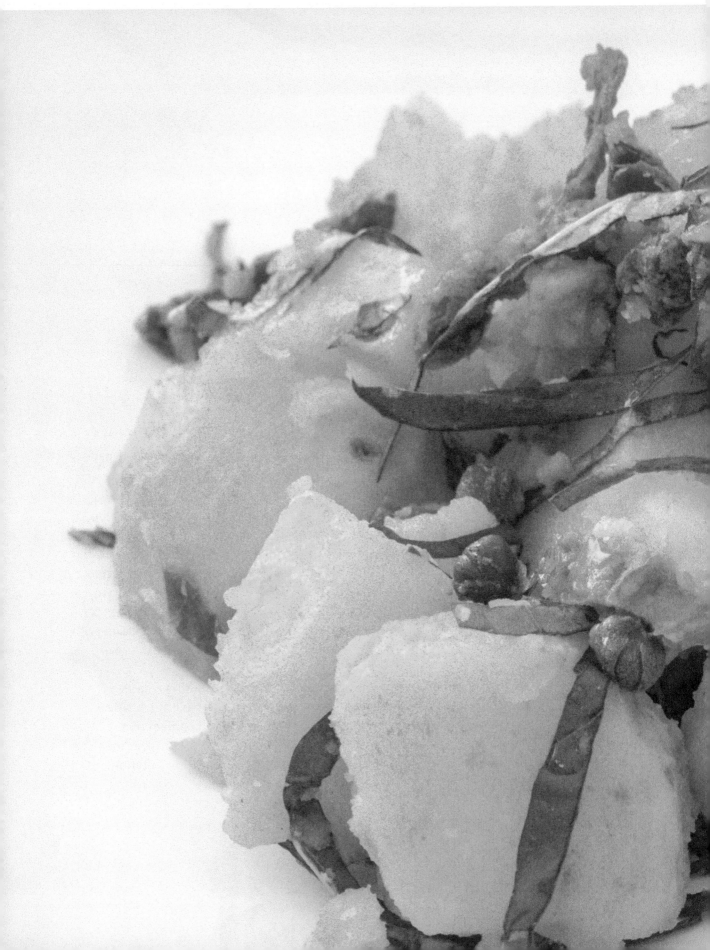

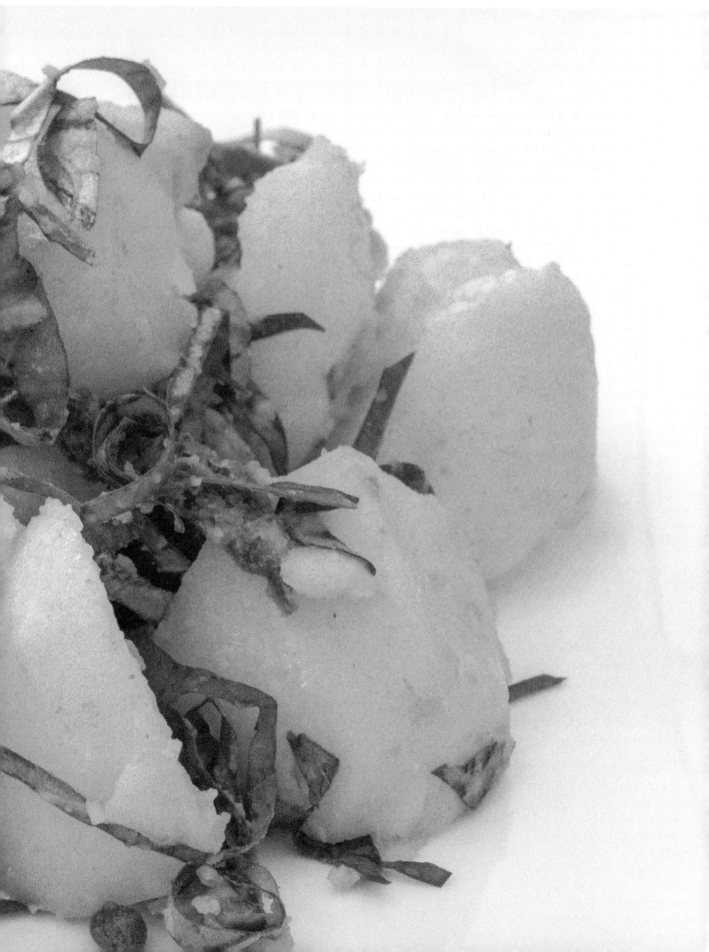

Saffron Potato Salad with Sun-dried Tomatoes

The use of saffron in this dish makes a lovely looking potato salad but an added benefit is the antioxidant benefits of both saffron and turmeric – a powerful combination!

55 minutes prep time
makes 4 servings

Ingredients

- 1 pound waxy yellow-fleshed potatoes – peeled
- Pinch of saffron threads (about 20)
- 3 tablespoons olive oil
- ½ cup sage leaves cut into long strands
- 12 sun-dried tomatoes (not in oil)
- 4 tablespoons capers
- Juice from one freshly squeezed lemon
- ½-1 tablespoon turmeric to taste
- Salt and freshly ground black pepper to taste
- 3-4 tablespoons Sicilian lemon balsamic vinegar (or other white vinegar as preferred) for tossing at end

Directions

1. Cut the potatoes in quarters.
2. Put in a large pan with just enough water to cover them. Add the saffron. Bring them slowly to a boil and then turn down the heat.
3. Simmer slowly until tender for about 25 minutes. Be sure to take the time to cook the potatoes slowly or they will disintegrate in the water. Drain when done leaving them still moist. Do not shake them dry in the colander.
4. Combine the sun-dried tomatoes and rest of ingredients (except the balsamic vinegar) in a small bowl and whisk with a fork.
5. Pour over hot potatoes and serve warm.
6. Add a few more sage ribbons for garnish and a drizzle with a good white balsamic vinegar

Tip: If you prefer a "fresh taste" without oil, you can eliminate the olive oil and just use lemon juice at the end.

Pumpkin, Saffron and Orange Soup

A rich tasting soup with a surprising array of sweetness to it. Garnish with pumpkin seeds to give it additional texture and a bit of a "crunch."

1 hour prep time
makes 2 servings

Ingredients

- 1 large onion, diced
- 1 large pumpkin
- 2 carrots, diced
- 1 teaspoon saffron fronds
- 2 teaspoon grated orange zest
- 2½ cups vegetable broth
- Salt and pepper to taste

Directions

1. Preheat the oven to 400 degrees.
2. Line a baking sheet with parchment paper and roast the pumpkin for 45-50 minutes or until soft to the touch. Scoop the roasted pumpkin from inside of shell.
3. Sauté the onion in a non-stick pan until soft and beginning to turn golden brown.
4. Add the pumpkin, carrot and saffron and stir together. Add the vegetable broth and bring to a boil. Lower the heat and simmer for about 15 minutes. Add the orange zest and simmer for five minutes longer.
5. Finish by processing the mixture with a food processor or Vita Mix. Add extra vegetable broth if the soup is too thick. Season to taste and enjoy!

Tip: You can also substitute butternut squash for this recipe as well.

Roasted Lemon and Herb Salad

The wonderful combination of flavors in this salad will be remembered long after you've tasted them. The contrast of sweetness and savory against its freshness is a real treat – especially during in the winter months when root vegetables are mostly available and used in recipes. Search out the finest and most colorful small tomatoes insuring the eye appeal of this wonderful salad.

25 minutes prep time
makes 4 servings

Ingredients

- 2 medium lemons sliced thin
- 1 teaspoon date sugar
- ½ teaspoon olive oil if preferred – otherwise you may leave the oil out of the recipe
- 8-10 sage leaves, cut in thin strips
- 1 cup small red cherry tomatoes
- 1 cup small yellow tomatoes
- 1 cup small orange tomatoes
- ½ cup flat leaf parsley leaves
- ½ cup fresh mint leaves
- 2 tablespoons pomegranate molasses
- Small red onion sliced thinly
- Salt and pepper to taste

Directions

1. Preheat the oven to 350 degrees.
2. Prepare the lemon slices for roasting by first bringing water to a boil in a small saucepan. Drop the slices in very hot water for about 2 minutes. Remove and drain well. Place the lemon in a bowl and toss with the date sugar and oil (if oil is preferred). Mix together well and place on a baking sheet lined with parchment paper.
3. Roast in the oven for about 15 minutes or until you see the lemons have dried out a little. This process will intensify the taste of the lemon. Over roasting will turn them black so watch them carefully.
4. When the lemons are done roasting combine all ingredients except salt and pepper in a large bowl. Toss together, add salt and pepper to taste.

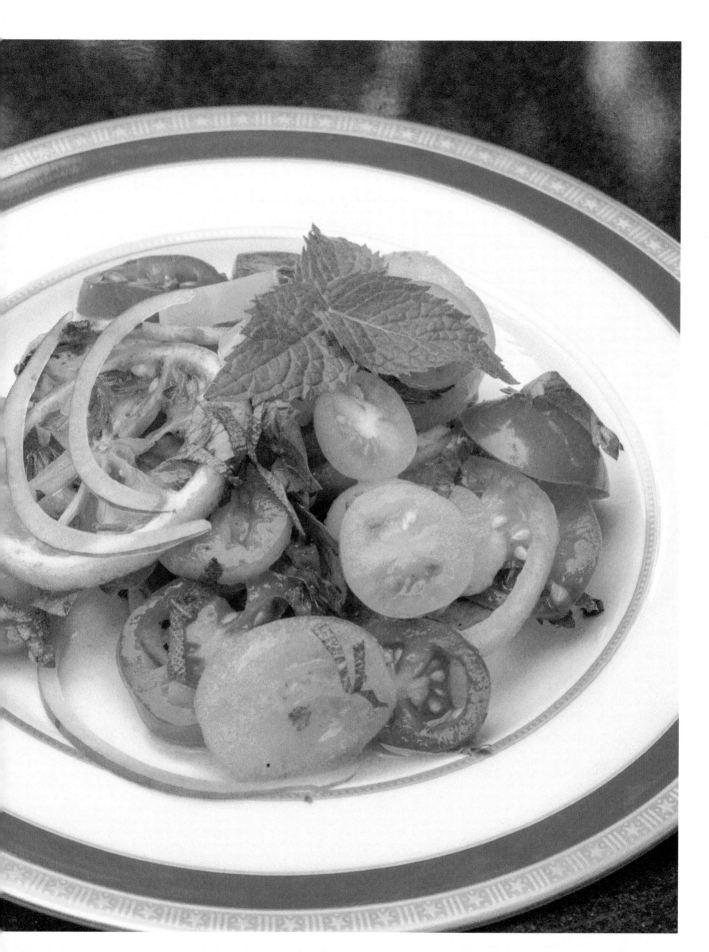

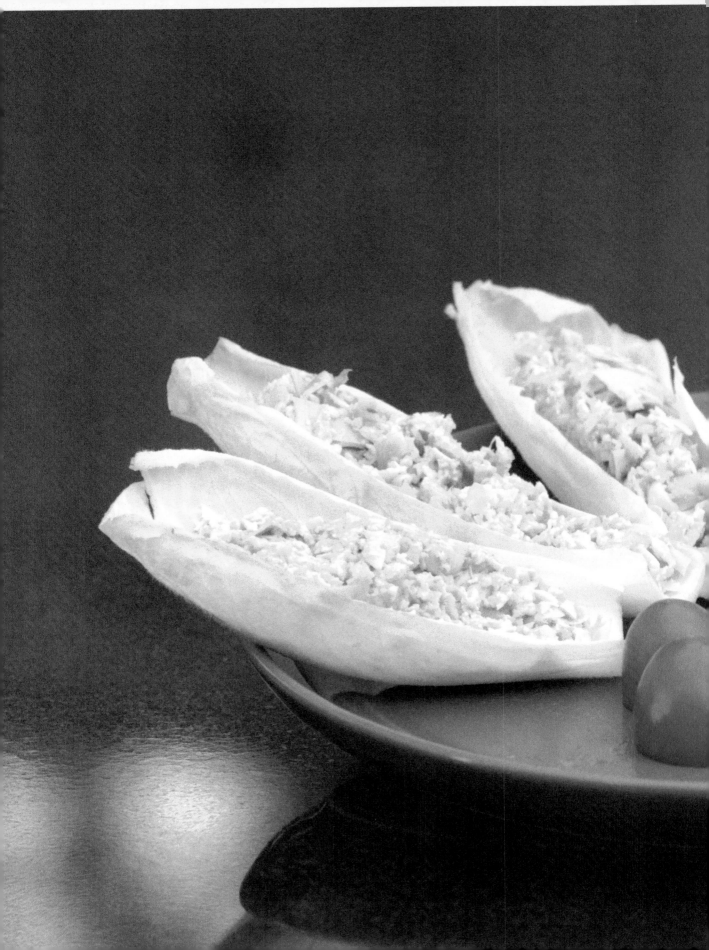

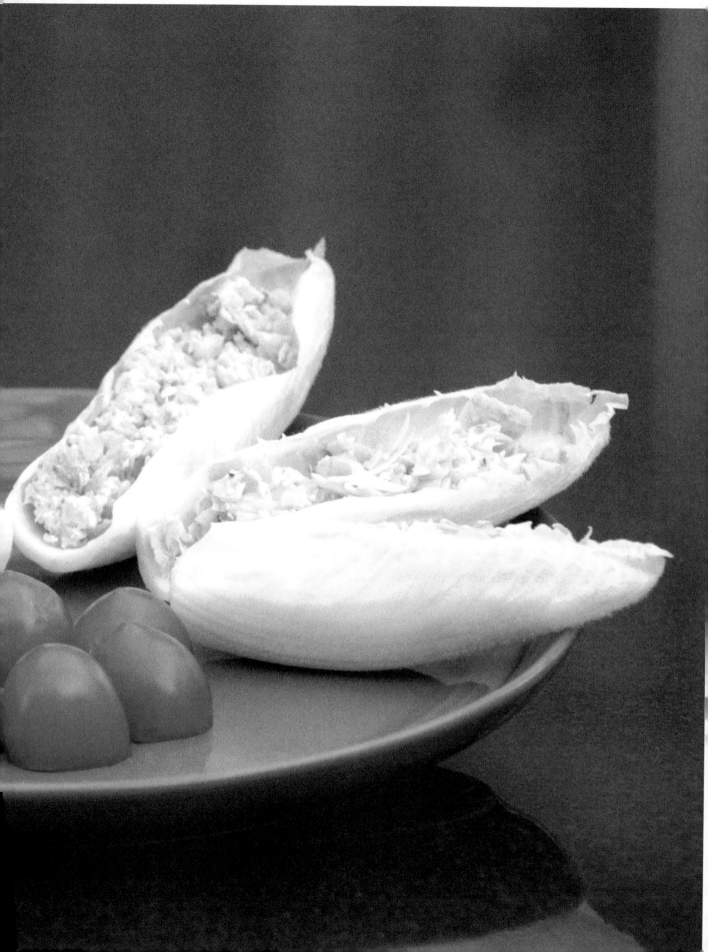

Artichoke and Walnut Stuffed Belgian Endive

When making this recipe be careful to not process the ingredients too much or you will end up with a pâté instead of a stuffing. I love getting the nutritional value of artichokes in unique ways such as this.

15 minutes prep time
makes about 12 pieces

Ingredients

- 15 ounce canned, fresh or frozen artichoke hearts, quartered
- ½ cup walnut pieces
- 3 cloves of garlic, crushed
- 4 tablespoons green onions, chopped
- Freshly ground black pepper
- 1 tablespoon olive oil (optional)
- 2 teaspoons fresh lemon juice
- ½ teaspoon minced thyme
- 3 medium Belgian endives, leaves separated
- 5 or 6 red grape or cherry tomatoes (for garnish)

Directions

1. If using frozen artichokes, cook until tender (about 10 minutes) in a medium saucepan. Drain and set aside. If using canned artichokes drain the liquid and set aside.
2. In a food processor combine the walnuts, garlic, green onions and pepper and process until chopped.
3. Add the oil (if using), lemon juice, thyme and artichoke hearts and mix together.
4. Scoop out artichoke mixture with a tablespoon and place on each opened endive leaf.
5. Arrange the filled endive leaves in a circular pattern and place red cherry or grape tomatoes in the middle.

Tip: As much as I like using fresh produce, using frozen or canned for this recipe really saves on time and work.

Delicious Kale Salad

A great salad that is filling and nutrient packed!

10 minutes prep time
makes 2 servings

Ingredients

- ½ bunch of kale (this recipe works well with Chouvert Frise kale)
- Handful of sunflower seeds (roasted but not salted) or pine nuts
- Dried cranberries to taste
- 4-5 tablespoons (or to taste) white balsamic vinegar or Sicilian Lemon Balsamic if available
- Small amount of honey for drizzling
- Small amount of olive oil for drizzling (optional)

Directions

1. Wash the kale and chop lightly. Do not cut it too small.
2. Arrange in a salad bowl and add nuts and cranberries.
3. Toss the ingredients together and add the balsamic vinegar.
4. After the salad is tossed drizzle honey and the optional oil on top.

Tip: There are a couple of variations you can make. You can substitute dried cranberries with fresh figs in this salad for additional nutrients of potassium and fiber. Another version is to substitute the sunflower seeds or pine nuts with roasted hazelnuts. Wonderful tasting!

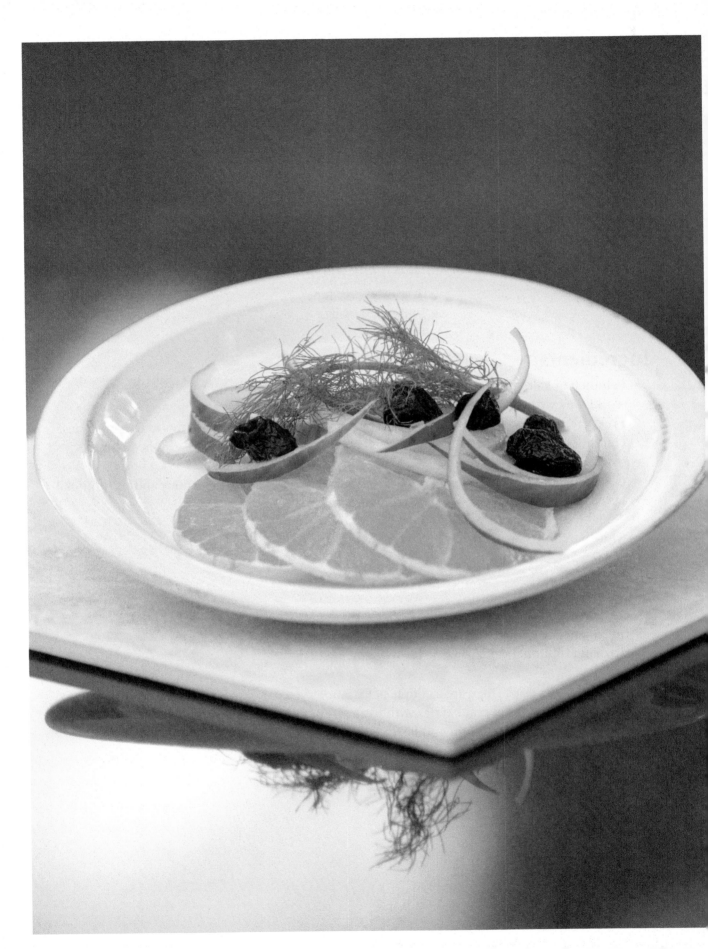

Fennel and Orange Salad

This salad has the flair of both Arab and Sicilian influence with its combination of citrus and olives. It's a staple in most households in Sicily.

10 minutes prep time
makes 2 servings

Ingredients

Salad
- 2 large oranges (navel oranges work and if you can find blood oranges, that's even better yet)
- 1 head of young fennel, preferable with green tops
- 1 red onion, sliced thin
- Sicilian black olives, dry cured

Dressing
- Fresh juice squeezed from one orange (in addition to the two oranges above)
- Pinch of sea salt
- 1 Tablespoon olive oil (optional)

Directions

1. Remove the peel of the two oranges and also cut off the bitter pith as well.
2. Cut off a small slice of the top and bottom of the orange. Using a sawing motion with a sharp serrated knife slice the orange in into thin rounds.
3. Finely slice the bulb of the fennel lengthwise and also cut the fine green tops of as well to use as garnish.
4. Finish by drizzling with the fresh squeezed orange juice, salt to taste, and the olive oil if desired.

Tip: It is important to buy a good quality balsamic vinegar for any of these recipes.

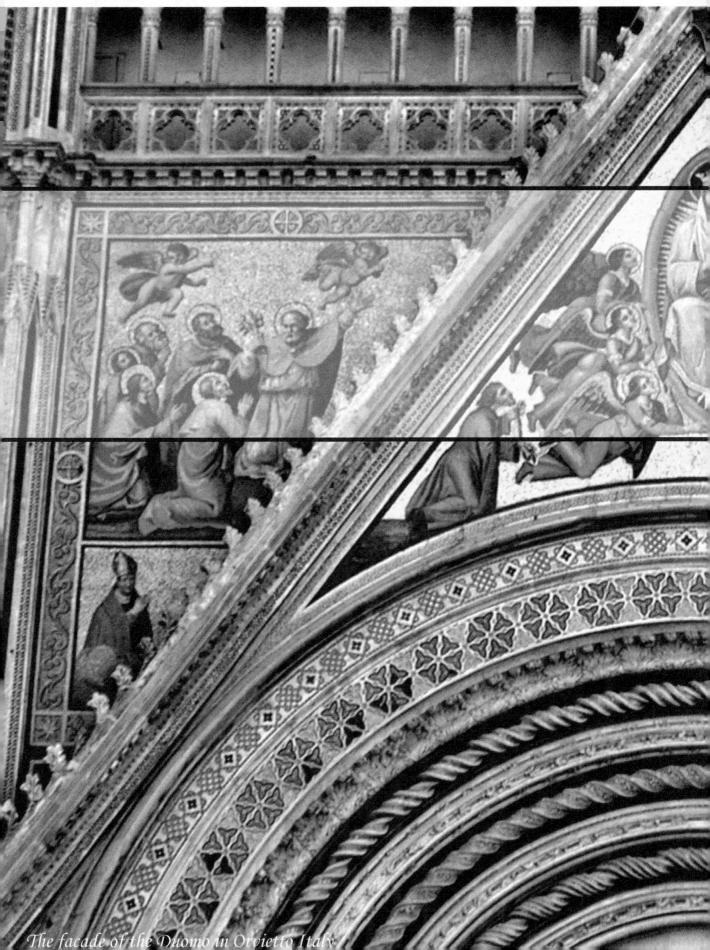

The facade of the Duomo in Orvietto Italy

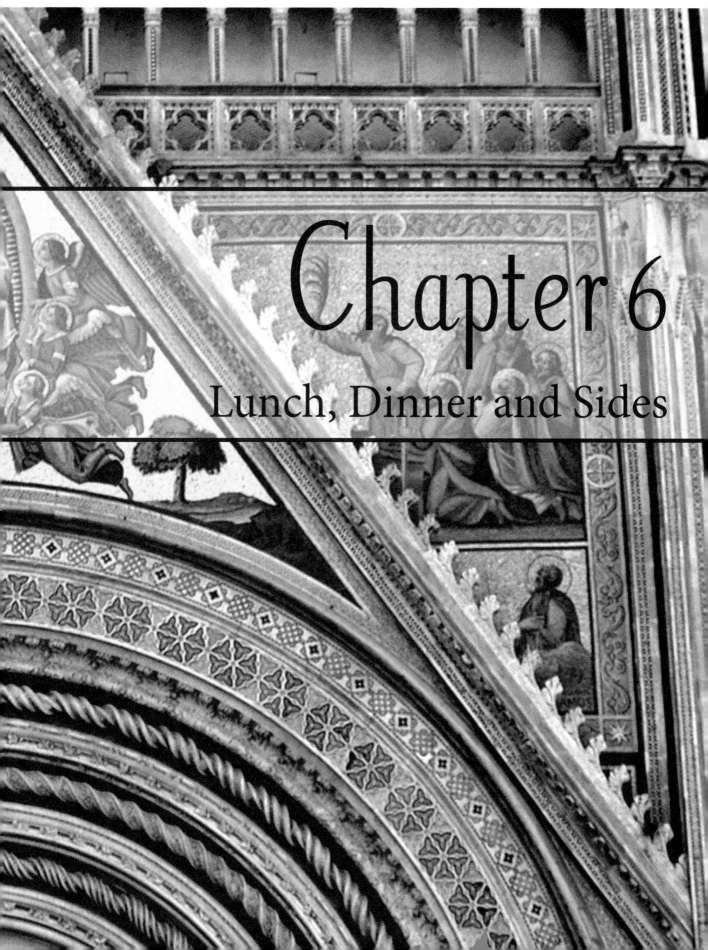

Chapter 6
Lunch, Dinner and Sides

Delicata Squash Rings with Fennel and Apple Relish

This is always a favorite of my students and I only use this recipe in the fall classes when temperatures are cool and delicata squash is in season. Choose squash that is firm to the touch with green markings on yellow skins

35 minutes prep time
makes 2 servings

Ingredients

- 2 delicata squash
- ½ cup dried cranberries
- 1 sweet crisp apple, washed well and diced
- 1 small fennel bulb, diced with outer layer removed
- ½ cup red wine, Madeira or port works well

Directions

1. Preheat the oven to 400 degrees and line a baking sheet with parchment paper.
2. Slice the ends off the squash and remove the seeds. Without peeling the squash slice it into ¾-1" rings.
3. Arrange the rings into a single layer and bake for about 30 minutes or until they are browned on the edges and the rings are softened enough to eat with a fork. Turn the rings half way through baking to brown both sides. The baking time will vary depending on how thick or thin you cut the rings and on how fresh the squashes are because squash toughens after storing for long periods of time.
4. While the rings are baking, combine all remaining ingredients in a small saucepan and heat (medium high) until the apple is softened and the liquid is absorbed.
5. Spoon over the rings right before serving and enjoy!

Tip: If you would rather not use red wine you can always substitute apple cider vinegar.

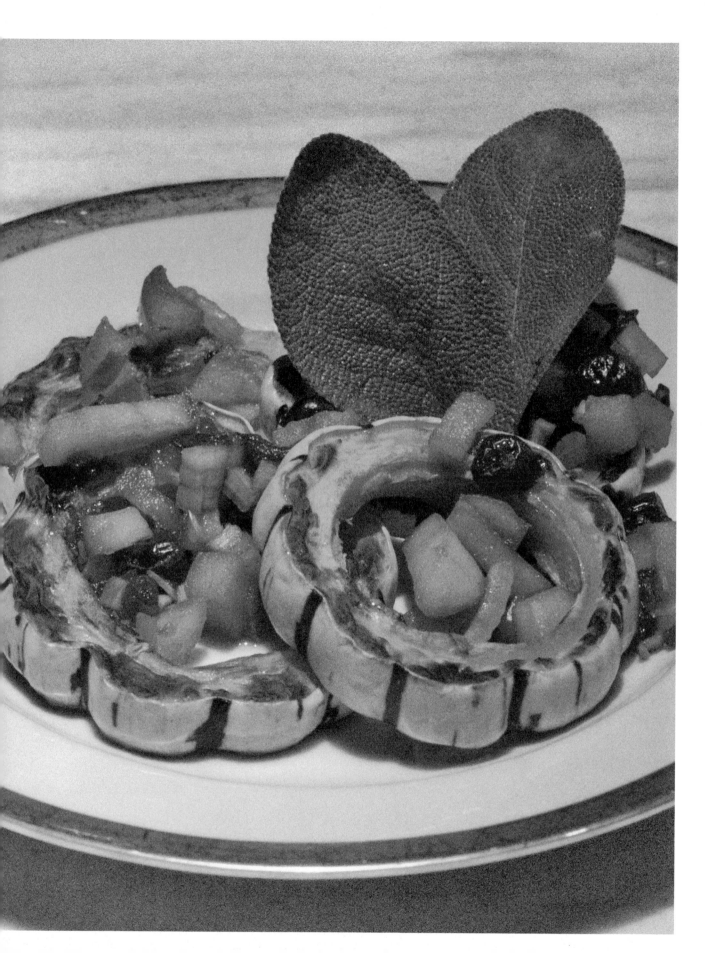

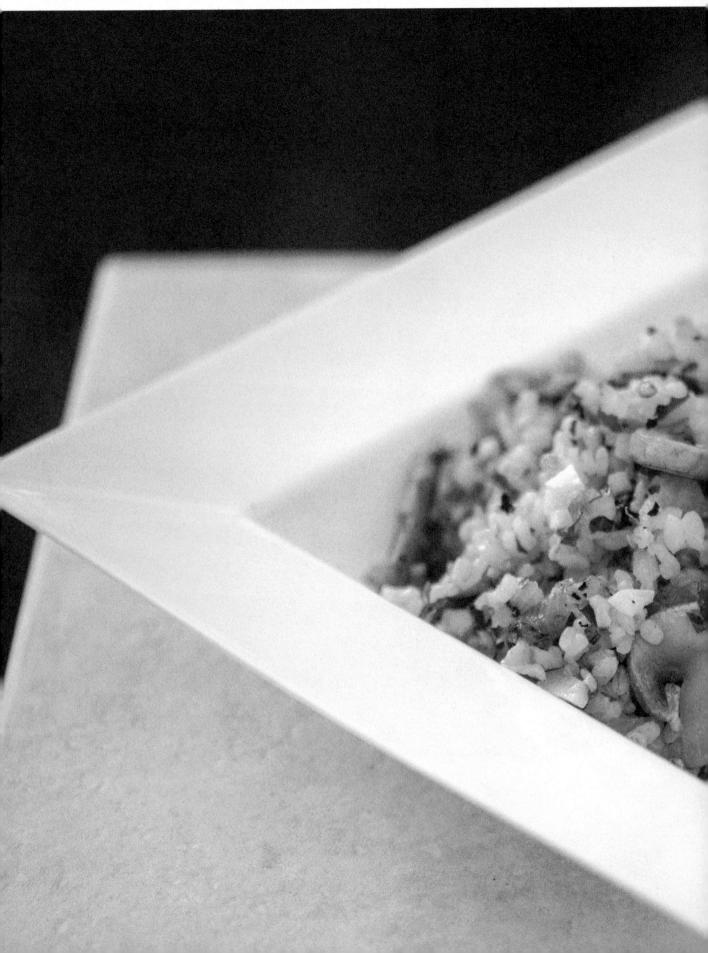

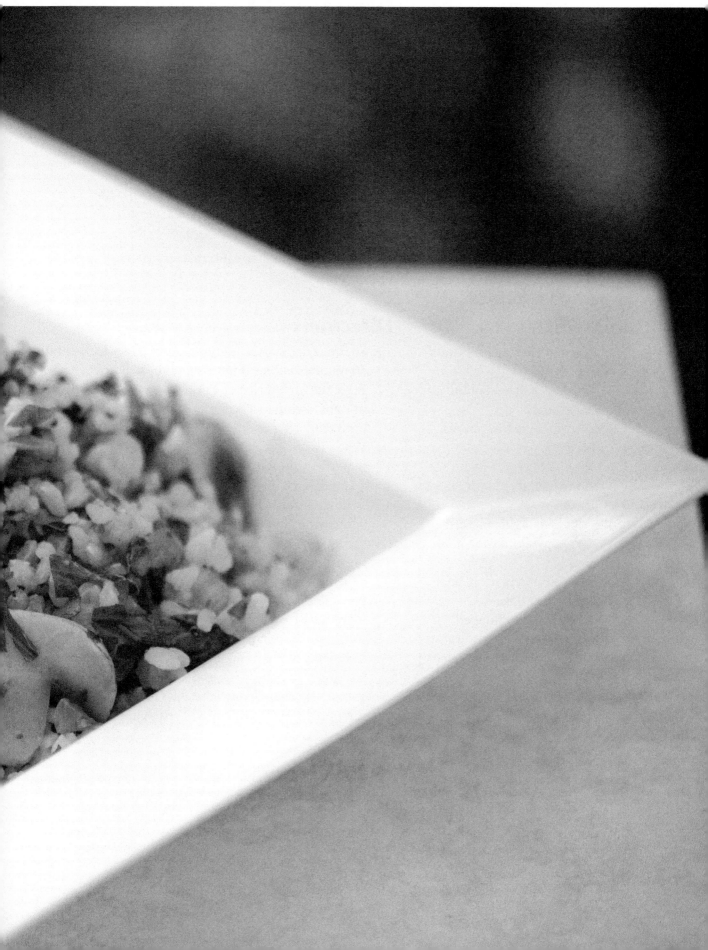

Brown Rice Risotto

If you are a risotto lover but miss it because you have eliminated white rice from your diet then this one is for you. In fact, once you make it you probably won't want to go back to the starchy white rice again.

45 minutes prep time, see tip below about shortening time
makes 4 generous servings

Ingredients

- 2 cups of short grain brown rice
- 2 ounces of dried porcini mushrooms
- 1 or 2 large yellow onions, diced
- 1 pound of asparagus, trimmed and cut into 1½ inch pieces
- 3 cloves of garlic, minced
- ¼-½ cups white wine if desired
- Fresh ground black pepper
- Red pepper flakes
- ⅓ cup parsley, chopped coarsely (you can also substitute chopped fresh rosemary)

Directions

1. Soak the dried porcini mushrooms in warm water for 30 minutes but keep the water after soaking.
2. Place the brown rice in a heavy pan and cover with 2" of water. Bring to a boil, stir once, cover and simmer until tender for about 35-45 minutes.
3. While the rice is steaming, begin sautéing all the other ingredients in a large pan except the red pepper flakes and parsley. For the liquid add small amounts of the soaking water from the mushrooms and a splash of white wine. Start with the onions as they will take the longest, then add the asparagus, garlic and rest of ingredients.
4. When the rice is still "al dente" remove it from the pan and place it in the large frying pan with rest of the ingredients.
5. Continue sautéing everything together while stirring frequently and adding liquid (the rest of mushroom soaking water and wine as needed) until the rice is completely coated and vegetables are infused within the rice. Top with parsley and red pepper flakes to taste.

Tip: In order to shorten the cooking time you can soak your rice in warm water for at least an hour before cooking. It will steam nicely in 15 minutes then. It's important to use short grain rice because it sticks together to make a great risotto, and long grain rice will not produce the same dish.

Delicious Lentils and Greens

I love the combination of flavors and textures in this high protein dish. The lentils serve almost as a background for the pop of flavor of the olives, the fresh taste of the tomatoes and the oregano adds a wonderful savory flavor to it all. It's quick to prepare and keeps well to enjoy the next day as well.

20 minutes prep time
makes 4 servings

Ingredients

- 1 cup green lentils (sometimes called French Lentils)
- 1 pint cherry or grape tomatoes
- Very large bunch of spinach (can also use Arugula or other green in place of spinach)
- Chopped fresh oregano to taste
- Black or Kalamata olives, cut in half
- Salt and pepper to taste
- ¼ cup or to taste balsamic vinegar

Directions

1. Rinse the lentils and place in a medium cooking pan. Add water to cover the lentils to about 1" above the top of the lentils.
2. Bring to a boil, stir once and reduce the heat to a simmer. Loosely cover the pan, stir occasionally and cook for about 18-20 minutes or until tender.
3. When the lentils have about 3-4 minutes left to cook (you will be able to tell by testing for doneness) add the spinach and let it steam in the pan with the lentils.
4. When finished, remove from the heat and add rest of ingredients, toss together with the balsamic vinegar at the very end and enjoy!

Tip: Fig, Vincotto or traditional Aceto balsamic all work well. Whichever vinegar you choose make sure you buy a good quality balsamic vinegar.

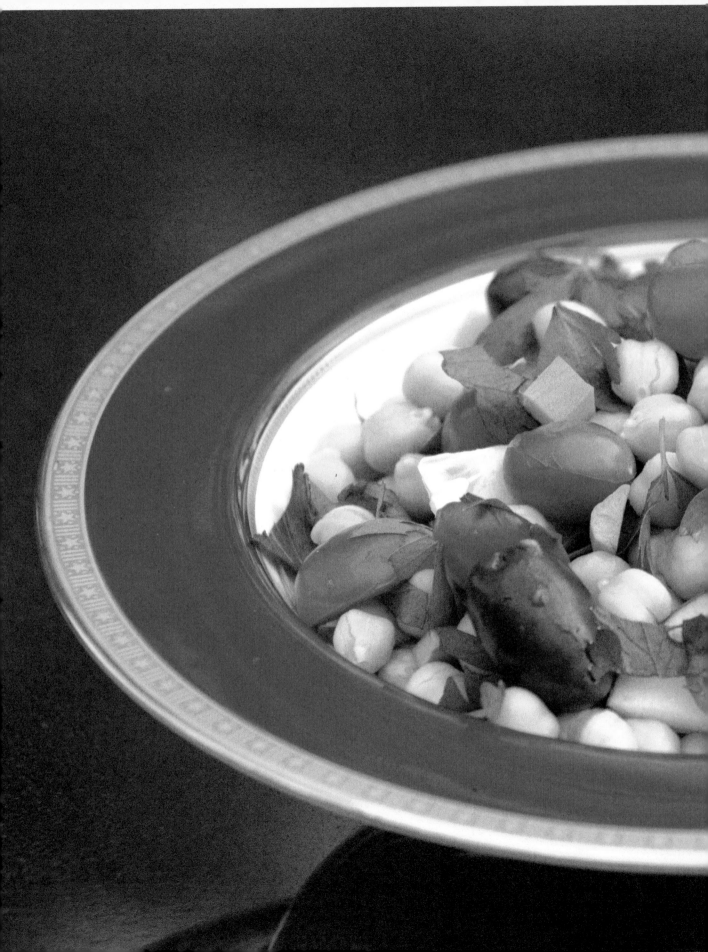

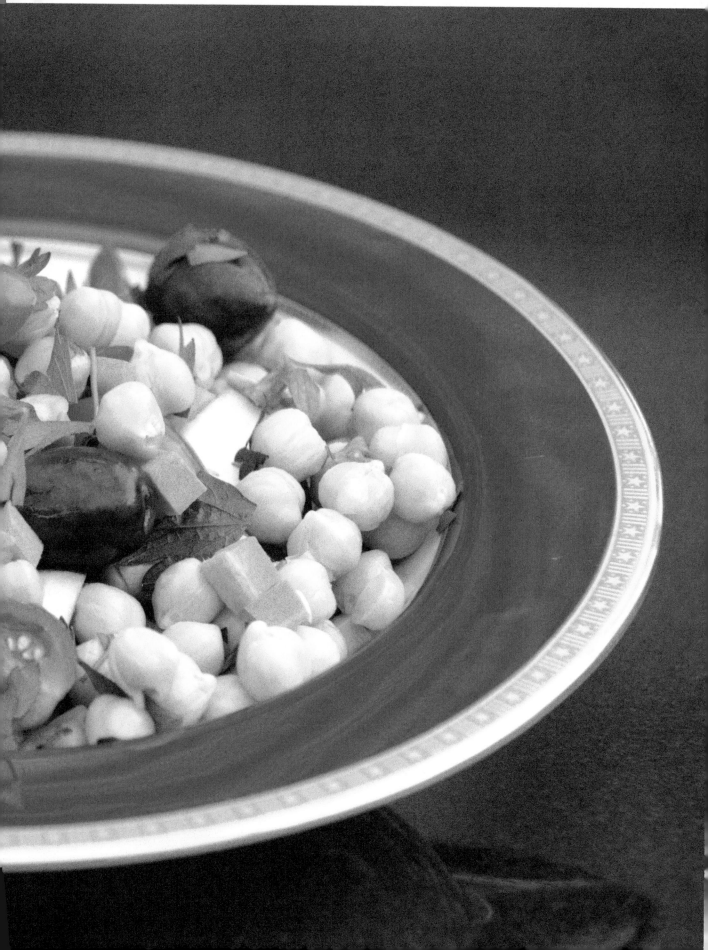

Garbanzo Bean Medley

This salad is delicious in the middle of summer when fresh tomatoes and produce is available and it's also great in the winter as a salad addition to a heartier meal.

25 minutes prep time
makes 2 servings

Ingredients

- 1 15 ounce can of garbanzo beans or 15 ounces of dried garbanzo beans that have been soaked overnight and simmered for about 30 minutes or until tender
- 1 cucumber, cut in ¼" slices
- 1 cup of grape or cherry tomatoes
- 1 large carrot, cut in ¼" slices
- 8 pitted kalamata olives, cut in half
- Small bunch of flat parsley, chopped
- White balsamic vinegar

Directions

1. Preheat the oven to 350 degrees.
2. Spread the tomatoes evenly on the bottom of a roasting pan that is lined with parchment paper. Lightly roast the tomatoes for about 15 minutes. If you have a convection feature on your oven, roast on convection for the last 5 minutes.
3. Toss all ingredients together adding the vinegar to taste, but reserve the chopped parsley and white balsamic vinegar.
4. Top with chopped parsley to garnish and white balsamic vinegar to taste.

Tip: Sicilian Lemon balsamic vinegar is a wonderful taste to this recipe if you can find it.

Pecan, Quinoa and Cranberry Stuffed Acorn Squash

This is a hearty fall and winter dinner entrée. The blend of sweetness from the cranberries with the savory of the shallots is just right!

1 hour prep time including roasting
makes 2 servings

Ingredients

- 1 large acorn squash, cut in half and seeds removed
- 1 large shallot, diced
- ½ cup cooked quinoa
- ¼ cup chopped pecans (you may want more if you like a crunchy texture)
- ¼ cup dried cranberries
- White balsamic vinegar to taste

Directions

1. Preheat the oven to 350 degrees.
2. Place the acorn squash halves cut side down on a pan with a little bit of water at the bottom. Bake the acorn squash halves until tender, usually about 45 minutes. The time can vary based upon the size and freshness of the squash
3. Sauté the shallot in a nonstick pan such as a Scan Pan that is safe to use.
4. Stir in the pecans, quinoa and cranberries.
5. Stuff the acorn squash with the quinoa mixture and bake an additional 10-15 minutes. Serve with a sprinkle of balsamic vinegar on top.

Tip: I used Sicilian Lemon balsamic vinegar. It's a favorite. Do use a white balsamic to avoid turning your beautiful recipe brown.

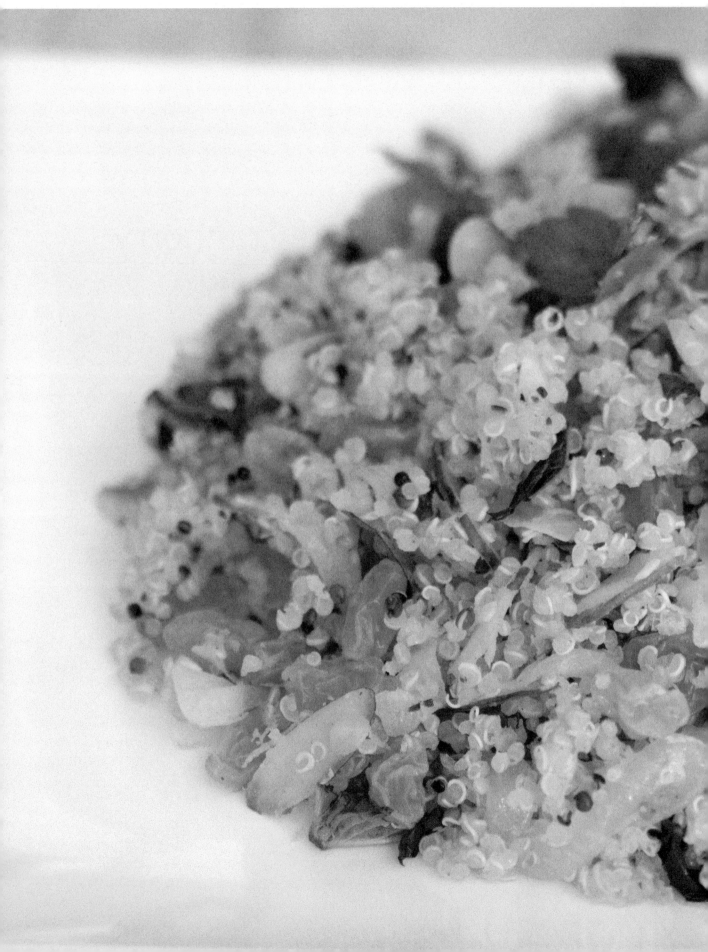

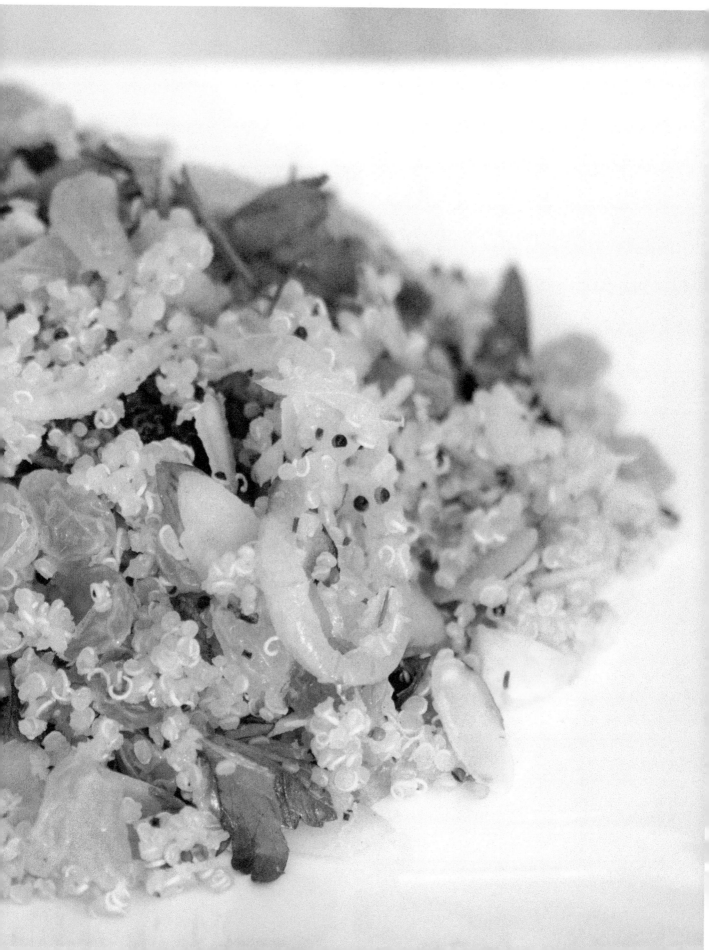

Moroccan Style Quinoa

This Moroccan inspired dish with its raisins, almonds, herbs, black cumin spice plus the addition of protein from quinoa makes it a perfect blend of taste and healthful nutrition.

18-20 minutes prep time
makes 2 generous servings

Ingredients

- 1 cup white quinoa
- 1 onion, sliced thinly
- ½ cup slivered almonds
- ½ cup golden raisins
- 3 cloves of garlic, roasted in their skin
- Small handful of flat parsley, chopped roughly
- 8 leaves of fresh mint, chopped roughly
- Zest of one organically grown lemon (or wash a conventionally grown lemon well)
- Juice of ½ lemon
- 1 teaspoon ground black cumin

Directions

1. Rinse the quinoa well. Place in a medium sized pan and cover with 2 cups of water. Bring the water to a boil, then lightly cover and simmer for 15–18 minutes or until the water is absorbed. Remove from the heat and fluff with a fork. The quinoa should be fluffy, not wet or overly cooked making it dry.
2. While the quinoa is cooking, place the thinly sliced onions in a nonstick pan (not Teflon or a coated pan) and sauté until they are caramelized. You will need to turn them often so they brown on all sides.
3. Gently toss the onions, quinoa and the rest of ingredients (except for lemon juice) together to combine. Sprinkle the lemon juice on top at the end.

Tip: If you've never roasted garlic before it's very easy to do and you will love the results. Start by placing the garlic cloves in a small fry pan. Do not remove the outer skin and do not add any oil to the pan. Roast using low to medium heat. Turn the garlic a few times to roast evenly. In about 10 minutes you will see the skins blacken which means the garlic is ready to use. Remove the skins and proceed with the recipe.

Zucchini Boats

This recipe makes a great dinner with a side of salad or rice or can serve as an appetizer when cut into four individual pieces.

30 minutes prep time
makes 4 servings

Ingredients

- 4 large zucchini, washed
- ¼ cup finely chopped vegan mozzarella cheese (if preferred, you could omit the "cheese" option)
- 2 tablespoons gluten free panko crumbs
- 16 cherry tomatoes
- 2 cloves garlic, finely chopped
- Fresh basil, chopped
- Salt and pepper to taste

Directions

1. Preheat the oven to 350 degrees.
2. Slice the zucchini vertically into two halves and make a slit from top to bottom on each of the halves.
3. Use a melon baller or a metal teaspoon measure and scoop out the insides of the zucchini until you have made a ¼ inch trough.
4. Place four cherry tomatoes inside each "zucchini boat" and sprinkle with garlic, cheese (if using) and bread crumbs.
5. Add salt and pepper to taste using just a pinch of salt.
6. Bake for 25 minutes or until the tomatoes are bubbly and the zucchini is tender when pierced with a fork.
7. Top with fresh chopped basil.

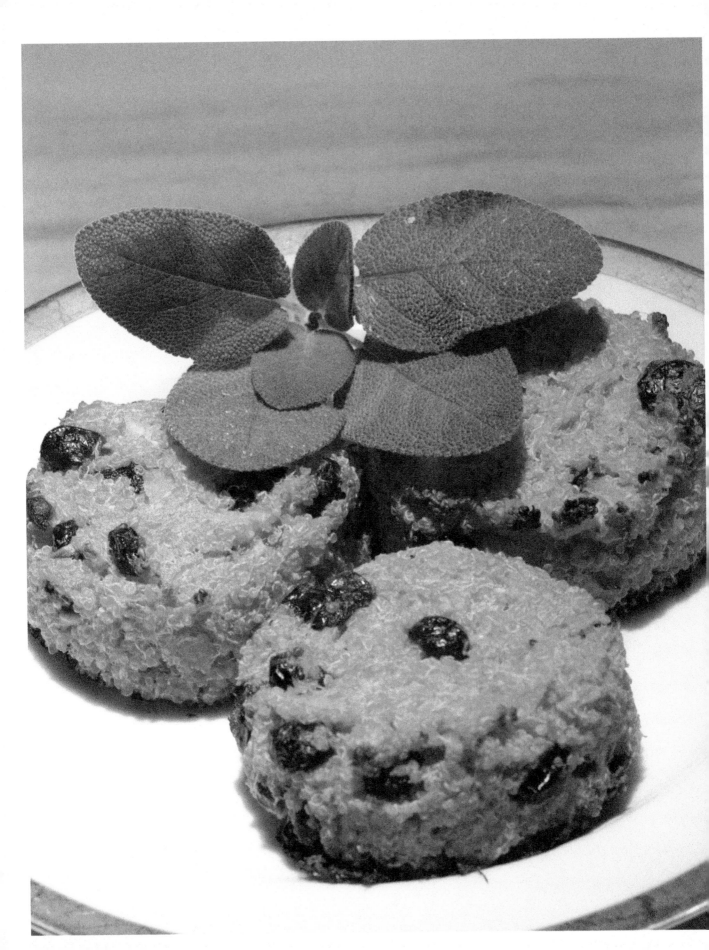

Sweet Potato Patties

These are delicious. I could eat them for breakfast, lunch or dinner. The tartness of the cranberries against the onion and vegetables is a wonderful combination of both sweet and savory.

1 hour prep time, mostly for roasting
makes 4 patties

Ingredients

- One large sweet potato, baked with inside removed and mashed
- 1 cup white quinoa
- ½ yellow onion, or two small leeks, finely sliced and diced (3-4 small green chopped onions also work, chop half way up the green part of the onion)
- 3 cloves of freshly crushed garlic
- Pinch of salt
- Fresh cracked pepper
- ¼ cup of dried cranberries or cherries
- 1 tablespoon apple or pomegranate juice (if needed to get correct consistency or desired sweetness)

Directions

1. Preheat the oven to 350 degrees and line a baking sheet with parchment paper.
2. Place the quinoa in a saucepan with 2 cups of water, bring to a boil, then simmer for about 15 minutes or until the quinoa is finished. Don't let it get too dry and finish by fluffing with a fork.
3. In a small saucepan slowly sauté the onion and garlic with the pinch of salt, stirring frequently. No oil is used in the pan so it keeps the flavors vibrant so that they are not masked with oil.
4. When the onions and quinoa are finished cooking, add all ingredients together in a large mixing bowl and stir well to combine.
5. Form the mixture into round balls and then flatten into a patty. If the mixture is too dry add a tablespoon of apple or pomegranate juice or you may want it for added sweetness.
6. Arrange the patties in a single layer and bake for about 45 minutes. The tops should be crispy and browned, and the bottom of the patties should be even more crispy. Don't over bake but be sure they are cooked through.
7. These can be served on a bed of lettuce, or accompanying roasted vegetables or just on their own.

Tip: These will keep well in the refrigerator for 3-4 days.

Indian Dosa

Dosa, a common food in Indian culture is rich in carbohydrates, and contains no sugar or saturated fats. Dosa can be used as crepes, a substitute for bread, as a wrap or as a side dish. This recipe (adapted from Chef, Anupy Singla) is protein rich due to the ingredients of quinoa and lentils and is naturally gluten free. The fermentation process increases the vitamin B and vitamin C content. These require a little time to prepare but after you make them once it's relatively easy. You just need to plan ahead for the time needed for soaking and fermenting the batter.

6 hours soaking time and 6 hours for fermenting
makes about 8 servings

Ingredients

- 3 cups white quinoa
- 1 cup white lentils
- 1 teaspoon fenugreek seeds
- 2 cups water at room temperature; you may need a little more.
- Scant teaspoon salt

Directions

Rinse and Soak

1. Rinse the quinoa and fenugreek seeds and transfer to a large mixing bowl. Add enough fresh water to cover the ingredients. Set aside to soak at room temperature for 6 hours to overnight.

Process

1. After soaking, drain the above mixture and discard the water.
2. Place the mixture in a high speed blender or Vita Mix with 2 cups of water (at room temperature) and process. Continue to process adding additional water if needed until the mixture is completely smooth.
3. Transfer the batter to a large mixing bowl and add the salt.
4. Stir together using your hands as some say that stirring the batter with your warm hands rather than a cold metallic spoon helps with the fermentation process.

Directions, Continued

Ferment

1. Cover the bowl with a damp dish towel and set aside in a warm dry place for 6 hours or overnight to allow the batter to ferment. If it's cool in the house and you want to make sure you have ideal conditions for fermenting, heat the oven to 200 degrees for 10 minutes. Turn off the oven, wait 10 minutes and place the covered bowl in the oven.
2. You should end up with a batter that is thin, slightly bubbly and frothy. Make sure that you use a large bowl as the batter will expand as it ferments.

Cook

3. Heat a non-stick pan (something like a scan pan). Pour approximately ¼ cup of the batter into the center of the pan. Using the back of a ladle or large spoon spread the batter in a circular motion from the center toward the outside of the pan creating a thin, round crepe.
4. Cook for 1 – 2 minutes on each side until lightly browned and pulled away from the sides of the pan. Don't be discouraged if the first few are difficult to cook and turn. Sometimes it takes a few tries to get the temperature and cooking process down.

> Tip: You will have enough batter for experimenting. Extra Dosai (plural) will keep for 2-3 days in the refrigerator. Uncooked batter also keeps in the refrigerator for 2-3 days.

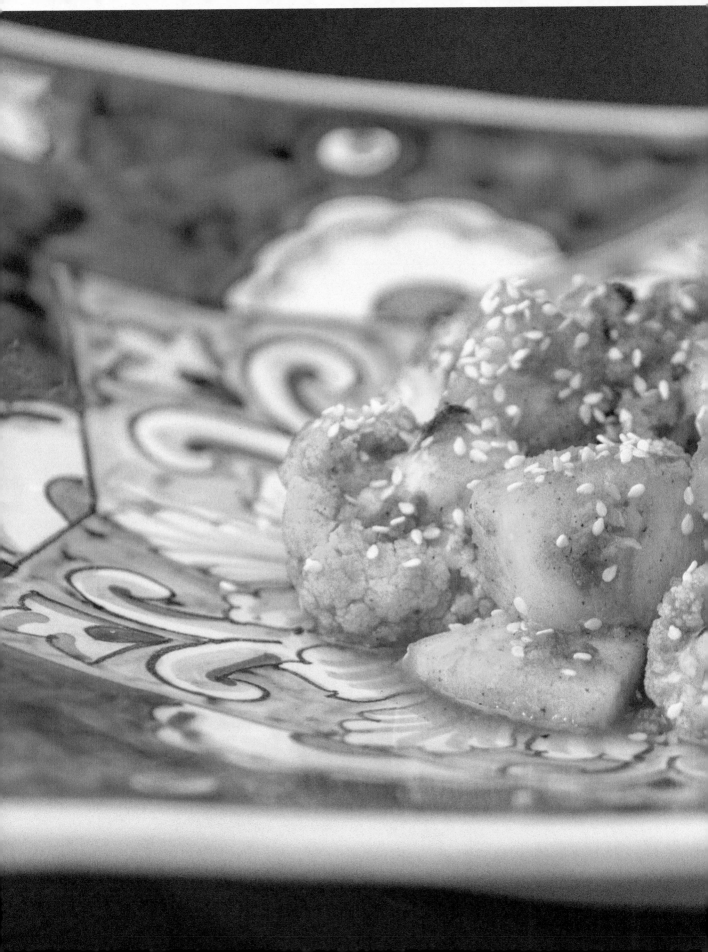

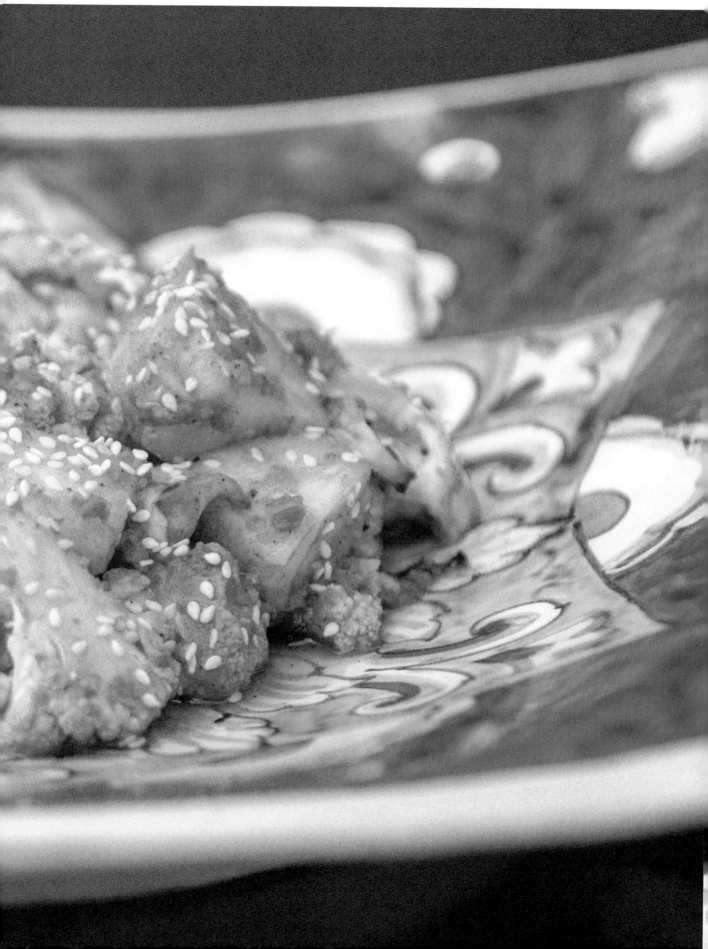

Sweet and Sour Pineapple Cauliflower

I've adapted this recipe from several others, one of which is from "I Could Never Be Vegan." The hot, spicy and sweet flavors deliver great taste. Both turmeric and cauliflower add high antioxidant value to this dish.

45 minutes prep time
makes 4 servings

Ingredients

- 1 head of cauliflower, separate the florets
- Turmeric, smoked paprika and fresh ground pepper, enough to sprinkle over the florets
- ⅓ cup finely diced fresh pineapple
- 1 cup fresh pineapple, not finely diced but chopped for the end of the recipe
- 2½ tablespoon sliced sundried tomatoes (not in oil)
- Juice of one lemon
- ½ cup water
- ⅓ cup white wine vinegar
- 4 tablespoons date sugar
- 1 tablespoon Braggs Liquid Aminos (or soy sauce)
- 1 tablespoon arrowroot flour (or cornstarch) mixed with a ¼ cup water
- ½ tablespoon hot Siracha sauce or more to taste if you like a spicy sauce
- ½ teaspoon ground ginger

Directions

1. Preheat the oven to 450 degrees.
2. Spread the cauliflower florets on a baking sheet that has been lined with parchment paper.
3. Sprinkle enough turmeric and fresh ground pepper to coat the cauliflower and toss to coat.
4. Roast the cauliflower until soft when pierced with a fork - usually about 20 minutes. Turn the florets over once insuring that they are roasted on both sides.
5. While the cauliflower is in the oven, make the sauce. Place the ⅓ cup finely diced pineapple, the sun-dried tomatoes and lemon juice in a food processor and process until smooth.
6. In a large shallow pan heat the water then add the vinegar, ginger, date sugar, soy sauce, Siracha. Add the pineapple and sun dried puree and cook over medium to low heat. When ingredients are combined, add the water and cornstarch mixture. Stir together and cook for another five minutes or until mixture has thickened. Add the reserved cup of fresh pineapple and combine the mixture with the roasted cauliflower making sure each piece is fully coated.
7. Sprinkle with sesame seeds and serve immediately.
8. This can be served alone as a side dish or over quinoa. Either way it is delicious!

Tip: To keep this dish vegan be sure to find a vegan brand because some Siracha sauces use anchovies as a base.

Quinoa-Stuffed Delicata Squash

This hearty dish is packed with fiber, nutrients and wonderful full-bodied taste. Be careful not to over bake them as they will get dry. The finished dish also keeps for another day or two in the refrigerator.

50 minutes prep time
makes 4 servings

Ingredients

- 2 delicata (or other squash as acorn, etc.) squash, cut in half length-wise with the seeds removed
- 1 teaspoon maple syrup
- 3 cups water
- 1½ cups quinoa
- 5 ounces baby arugula (I've also used spinach)
- ⅓ cup dried figs chopped
- ⅓ cup dried currants (optional)
- ⅓ cup dates pitted and chopped
- ½ cup roasted pumpkin seeds
- ½ teaspoon salt
- Fresh ground pepper

Directions

1. Preheat oven to 375 degrees and line a large baking sheet with parchment paper.
2. Brush maple syrup on to the flesh side of each squash and place them face down on the baking sheet. Roast for 20 minutes or just until tender. Let cool.
3. Meanwhile, bring water to a boil in a medium saucepan. Add quinoa, reduce to low heat and cover. Cook for 15-18 minutes or until all the water is absorbed. Turn heat off, and let sit for 5 minutes.
4. Remove cover, add arugula, figs, currants and dates to the pot. Replace cover and let sit for 5 minutes.
5. Transfer quinoa contents to a large bowl and fluff with a wooden spoon. Add ¾ of the pumpkin seeds and stir to coat. Season with salt and pepper to taste.
6. Fill each squash half with finished quinoa stuffing. Place each half in a 9x13 baking dish and cook for a remaining 20-25 minutes until warm.
7. Sprinkle with remaining pumpkin seeds on top. Serve and enjoy!

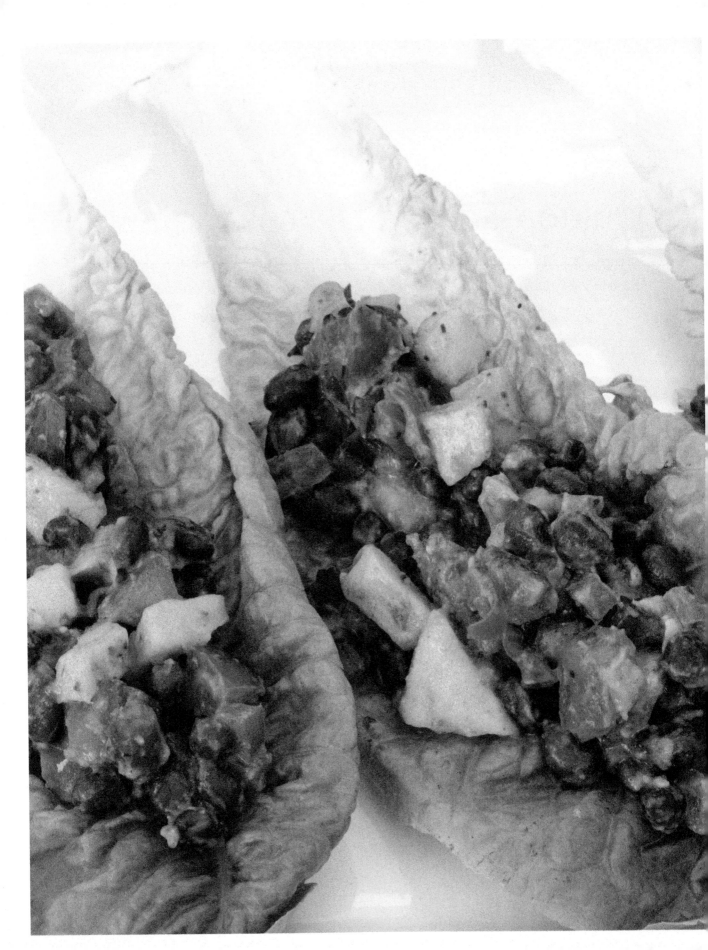

Black Bean and Mango Wrap

This quick and easy recipe is packed with flavor and nutritional value. The contrast between sweet, savory, heat and spice is pretty amazing – especially for how quickly it comes together.

10 minutes prep time
makes 4 servings

Ingredients

- 2 cups cooked black beans
- ½ large ripe avocado – peeled and pitted
- 4 cloves of roasted garlic
- 1/3 c fresh tomatoes, copped
- ½ medium green pepper, chopped
- 1 mango, diced
- 1 jalapeño pepper, diced
- 3 green onions, chopped (use part of the green stem as well)
- ¼ c parsley, chopped
- 2 T fresh lime juice
- 1 t ground cumin (use black cumin if possible)
- 1 t chipotle chili pepper or cayenne pepper
- 8 large romaine leaves

Directions

1. Mash the black beans, avocado and garlic together with a fork until well blended and slightly chunky. Add all ingredients except the lettuce and mix.
2. Place approximately ¼ cup of the mixture in the center of each lettuce leaf and roll like a burrito.

Cauliflower, Swiss Chard and Chickpea Dish

All the recipes for this book are healthful and this one is packed with high value nutrients with the cruciferous vegetable cauliflower, fiber and protein from chickpeas and antioxidants delivered through the addition of turmeric and cumin. To top it all off the taste is outstanding.

10 minutes prep time
makes about 8 pancakes

Ingredients

- 1 head of cauliflower, separated into large florets
- 1 teaspoon ground cumin
- 6 large Swiss chard leaves, cut into thick strips
- 1 red onion, cut into wedges on the thinner side
- 3 garlic cloves, chopped roughly
- 1 15 ounce can of chickpeas rinsed and drained (you can soak dried chickpeas and cook them if preferred)
- Fresh squeezed lemon juice from one lemon
- Sea salt and fresh ground pepper to taste

Directions

1. Heat a nonstick skillet or fry pan over medium heat and add the cauliflower florets. Cook for about ten minutes, or until the florets are a dark golden brown. Turn the florets often so they brown evenly and don't stick to the pan.
2. Add the cumin and toss together in the pan so the florets are evenly coated.
3. Add the Swiss chard, onion and garlic and cook together for a couple more minutes.
4. Add the chickpeas last and cook just long enough for the chickpeas to warm through.
5. Season with salt and pepper to taste.
6. Top with lemon juice and serve immediately.

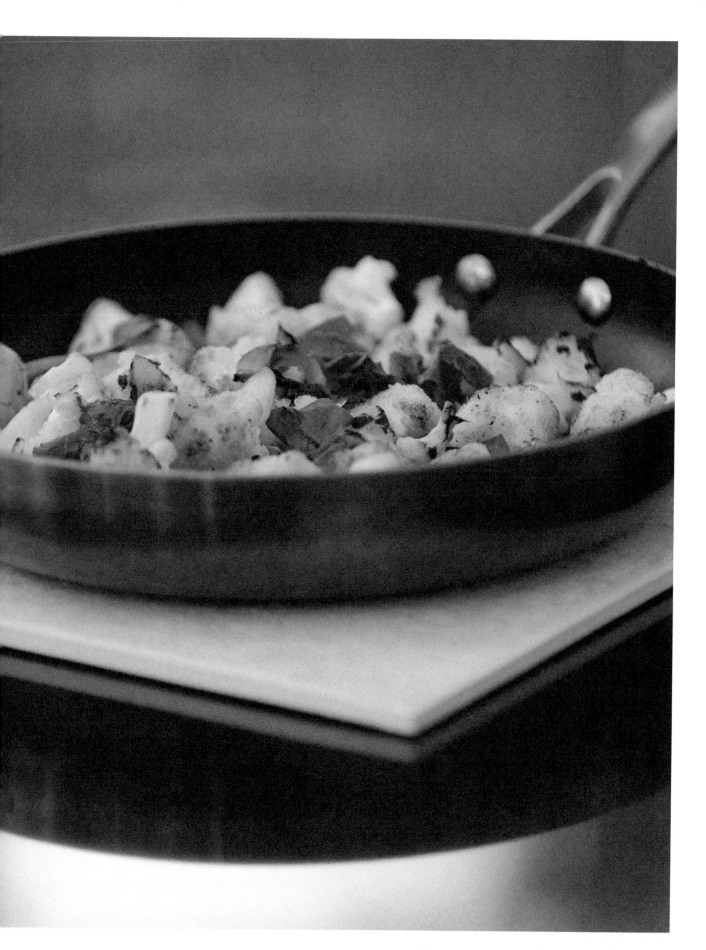

Spaghetti Squash with Spinach, Olives and Almonds

This dish turns out best when squash is in season and hasn't been stored too long, usually mid fall until December. The "spaghetti" is a perfect background for the combined flavors of the added ingredients.

about 1 hour prep time
makes 4 servings

Ingredients

- 4 pounds of spaghetti squash, whole
- ½ pound baby spinach
- ⅓ cup pitted black olives, chopped
- 1 tablespoon capers, chopped
- ½ cup almonds, chopped
- ⅓ cup fresh parsley, chopped roughly
- Sea salt and pepper to taste

Directions

1. Preheat oven to 350 degrees.
2. Place the whole spaghetti squash in the oven. You can place it directly on the oven rack to roast or place it on a parchment lined baking sheet. Let the squash roast turning once. Using oven mitts press the squash gently, when it's soft to the touch roasting is complete. Depending on the squash, it takes about 45 minutes to roast.
3. Once squash is cool enough to handle, use a fork to scrape spaghetti squash into a large bowl. It should separate easily and look like golden spaghetti.
4. Season spaghetti squash with salt and pepper to taste.
5. Add spinach into squash. Toss to evenly coat squash and greens. There is no need to steam the spinach first. It will gently steam while tossed with the hot spaghetti squash.
6. Add olives, capers, almonds and fresh parsley; toss to evenly distribute

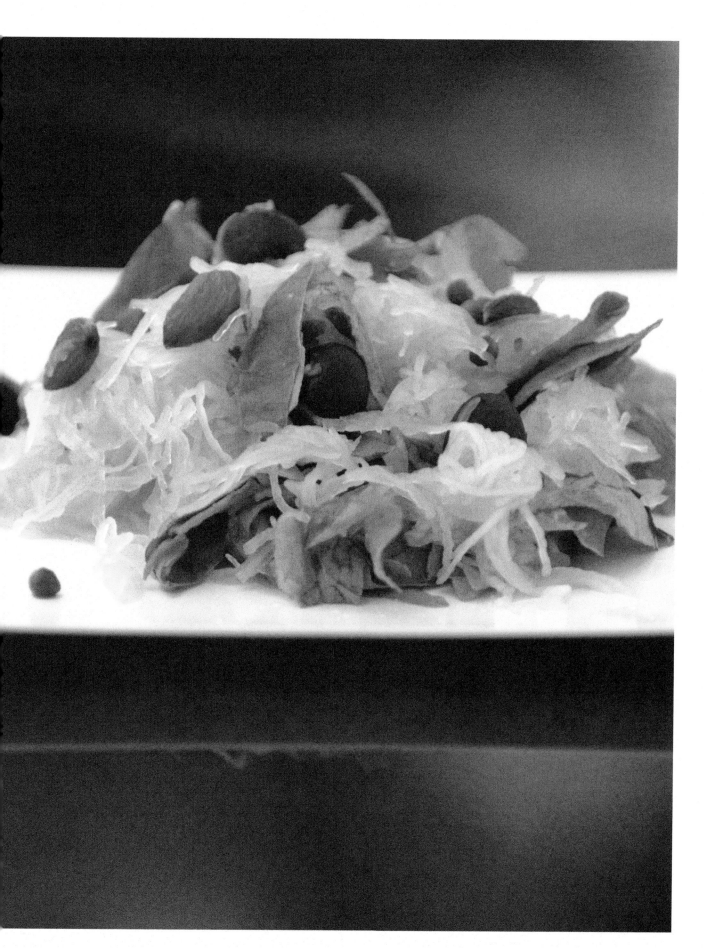

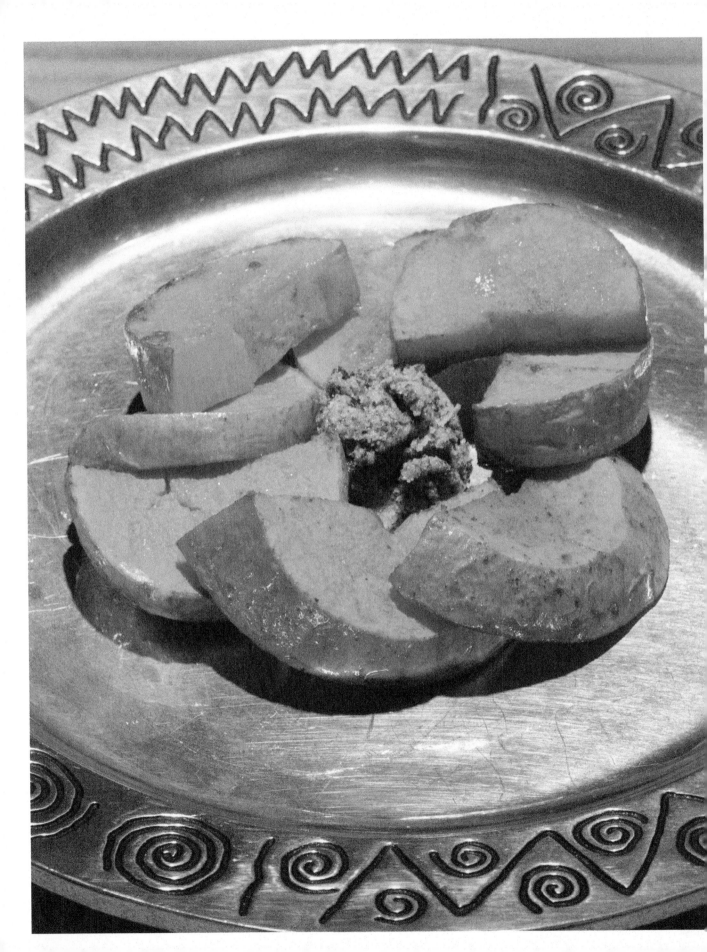

Roasted Butternut Squash Wedges

Elegant, delicious and a burst of wonderful flavors. I also made a walnut sage pesto for a dinner (shown in the middle of the dish) to accompany these wedges as we were hosting a dinner party. It is optional however as the squash is delicious on its own.

25 minutes prep time
makes 4 side servings

Ingredients

- 1 medium sized butternut squash
- 2-3 tablespoons brown or date sugar
- ¼ teaspoon salt
- 2-4 tablespoons cayenne or chili pepper to taste
- 1 tablespoon olive oil for tossing if desired.

Directions

1. Preheat the oven to 450 degrees and line a baking sheet with parchment paper.
2. Cut the butternut squash in half lengthwise and remove the seeds. Cut each of the halves of squash in half width wise, right where the slender part curves out to the bulge. Now cut 1" thick wedges and place in a large bowl.
3. Toss the wedges in the rest of the ingredients to coat well.
4. Place in a single layer on a baking sheet and roast for about 15 minutes or until browned on one side. Then turn over to roast on the other side. The wedges will caramelize on the edges and you will need to move them about the baking sheet so they don't stick.
5. Remove and place on a platter, ideally with a metal surface that will hold the heat.

Tip: If you would like to add the Walnut Sage Pesto shown in the picture see page 150 for the recipe.

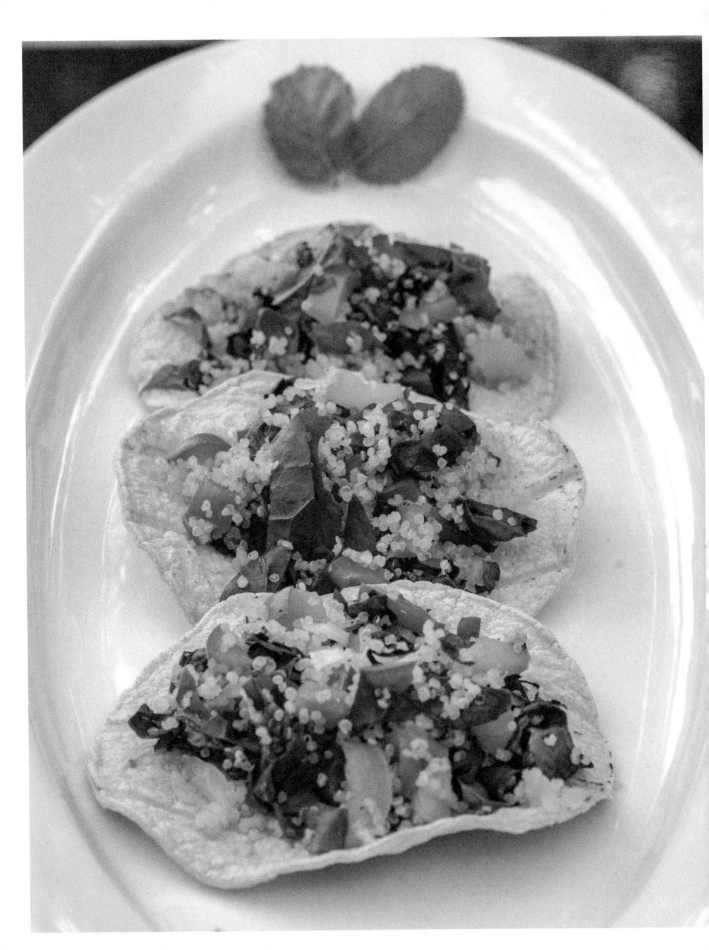

Caramelized Onion and Quinoa Tacos

I love using quinoa in various ways. It's among the most versatile grain available and works well in many cuisines. Here it's used as a background for the flavors of the onion and the texture and nutritional benefits of the swiss chard. I've also included sautéed red and yellow peppers for added flavor, color and nutritional benefits.

25 minutes prep time
makes 2 servings

Ingredients

- ½ cup white quinoa
- ½ yellow onion
- 2 cloves garlic minced (more or less to your taste preference)
- 3 cups swiss chard
- ½ teaspoon crushed red pepper
- 2 (non-GMO) corn tortillas or sprouted grain tortillas (Ezekiel brand is good)
- White wine balsamic vinegar

Directions

1. Preheat the oven to 350 degrees.
2. Place the tortillas directly on the oven rack and bake until crisp, about 5 minutes, and remove from the oven.
3. Rinse the quinoa well and place in a medium size saucepan. Cover with 1 cup of water. Bring it to a boil, stir once, then simmer for about 15 minutes or until the water is absorbed and the quinoa can be "fluffed" with a fork.
4. While the quinoa is cooking thinly slice the onion and sauté it in a non-stick pan (see equipment needs) turning occasionally until it begins to caramelized.
5. When the onion is soft and almost browned add the garlic and swiss chard. Cover and cook another 5 minutes or until the swiss chard is wilted.
6. Stir in the quinoa and crushed red pepper.
7. Fill the tortillas with the above mixture and drizzle with the white wine vinegar. If the tortillas aren't too crispy you can fold them and eat them but if they are too crisp to fold, enjoy them as an open faced sandwich.

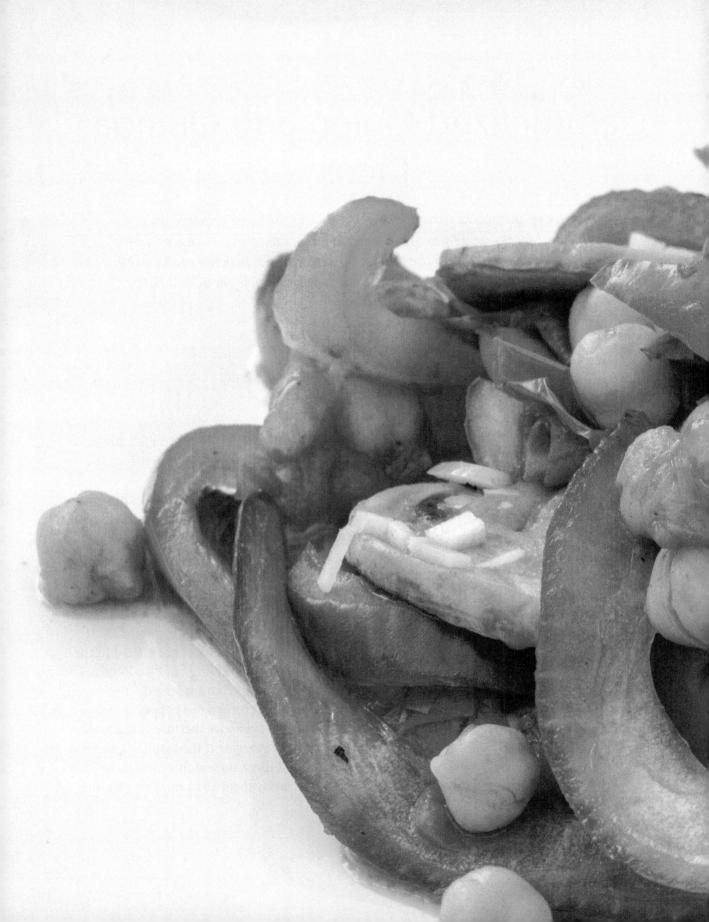

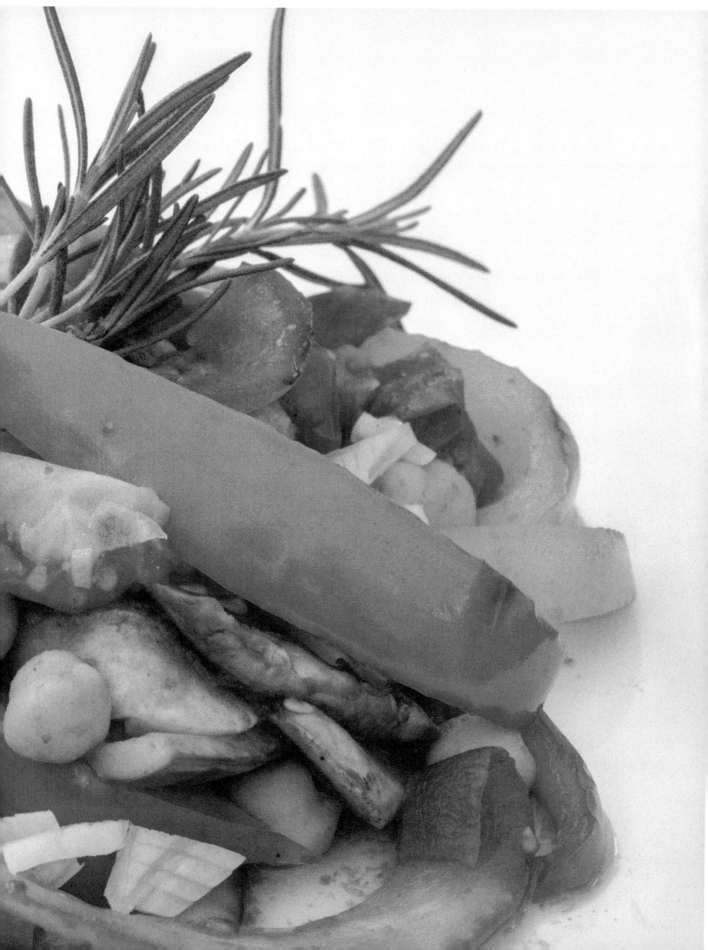

Roasted Chickpeas with Grilled Vegetables

The flavors of roasted vegetables and chickpeas come together nicely and the "pop" of flavor at the end from the Sicilian Lemon balsamic vinegar is a great combination. If you can't find Sicilian Lemon vinegar try good quality white vinegar. It adds a "pop" of flavor at the end.

45 minutes prep time
makes 3 generous servings

Ingredients

- 12 small mushrooms, sliced
- 2 ripe tomatoes, cut into quarters
- 1 red and yellow bell pepper cut in strips
- 1 red onion or 1½ cups leeks, cut into wedges
- About 6 cloves of garlic, un-peeled
- 4 cups of garbanzo beans (chickpeas) - either canned and rinsed well or purchased dried and cooked.
- 2 sprigs of fresh rosemary
- Balsamic vinegar to taste

Directions

1. Preheat the oven to 400 degrees if roasting in the house, or prepare a hot grill (preferred method for best flavor - see notes for grilling vegetables in chapter 2).
2. Put the mushrooms, tomatoes, red and yellow peppers, onion and garlic in a large roasting or grill pan. Roast for about 30 minutes or until you can see the vegetables caramelizing.
3. Remove the pan and turn the vegetables over. Add the chickpeas and rosemary and return to the oven or the grill pan. Roast for another 30-45 minutes until the edges of the vegetables are starting to turn dark and the chickpeas are browning.
4. Remove the skin on the garlic, mince and return to the mixture.
5. Sprinkle with balsamic vinegar, toss together and serve warm. This dish can be served on its own or over quinoa.

Tip: I prefer Sicilian Lemon from The Olive Tap if you have easy access to it, otherwise white wine vinegar will be a good substitute. As much as I try to avoid canned foods sometimes it's better to have them available than to miss the nutritional benefits of garbanzo beans.

The Perfect Nutrient Dense Wrap

This is my favorite wrap recipe. It's satisfying as a lunch and sometimes dinner with addition of a side of salad or fruit. It is "nutrient dense" and you can vary it with your favorite fillings or to reflect the vegetables you have at the time. Experiment a little. You might be surprised at what you can create.

20 minutes prep time
makes 2 wraps

Ingredients

- 4 tablespoons of hummus (see page 162)
- 2 green onions, chopped
- ¼-½ cup washed spinach, if using baby spinach there is no need to chop but if it's fresh spinach from the garden you should chop it into smaller pieces.
- About 6 sun dried tomatoes
- ½ red pepper, copped finely
- Sprinkle of balsamic vinegar (optional)

Directions

1. Preheat the oven to 450 degrees.
2. Lay two tortillas on a flat surface. Spread the tortilla generously with the hummus, at least two tablespoons per wrap.
3. Next, line the middle of the tortilla with chopped onions, then line with chopped red pepper and finally the sun dried tomatoes.
4. Top it all with lots of fresh spinach.
5. Sprinkle a thin line of balsamic vinegar across the spinach (this is optional - experiment a little).
6. Carefully roll into a burrito like roll keeping all ingredients together as you roll. If any spinach leaves have fallen out stuff them back into the ends of the wrap.
7. Put on a baking sheet and bake until all ingredients are heated through and the wrap is crisp. This takes about 10-15 minutes. Cut each wrap in half or into thirds depending on your preference and enjoy!

Tip: My favorite wrap uses Ezekiel's 4:9 sprouted grain tortillas. You can also use other brands of sprouted grains, corn tortilla, and whole wheat tortilla (if not gluten intolerant) or the leaves of lettuce, kale or collard greens as a base. You can also easily make your own hummus or you can buy hummus made with or without oil. Sahara Cuisine or Oasis Classic are two commercially made hummus made without oil but Cedar farms hummus is made with oil.

Roasted Artichoke, Lemon and Herb Dish

This is a hearty and filling side dish to complete any meal or it's wonderful as a main course with the addition of green vegetables. The flavors come together wonderfully!

1 hour prep time
makes 2 servings

Ingredients

- 2 pounds small red potatoes
- 2 cans of artichoke hearts
- 4 cloves garlic, crushed
- About 8 sage leaves, roughly chopped
- Fresh ground black pepper
- 2 lemons, sliced thinly
- 1 cup cherry tomatoes
- 1 cup Kalamata olives (without the pits)
- ½ cup parsley, roughly chopped

Directions

1. Preheat the oven to 400 degrees.
2. Wash the potatoes well (leave skins on) and place them in a large pan and cover with water. Boil for about 15 minutes or until half cooked.
3. Once half cooked, drain, cut in half and place on a large baking sheet lined with parchment paper and place them in the oven to begin roasting.
4. Roast for 20 minutes.
5. While the potatoes are roasting rinse the artichokes and cut in half if too large. Mix together with the lemon slices, Kalamata olives, garlic, sage and cherry tomatoes.
6. After the potatoes have roasted for 20 minutes, add the above mixture to the pan and continue roasting. Roast for another 20 minutes or until potatoes are browned. Stir once while roasting to insure that everything is browned on all sides.
7. Remove from the oven and garnish with the parsley.

Tip: You can always use fresh artichokes if you prefer, but the work of preparing them for the recipe is labor intensive and time consuming.

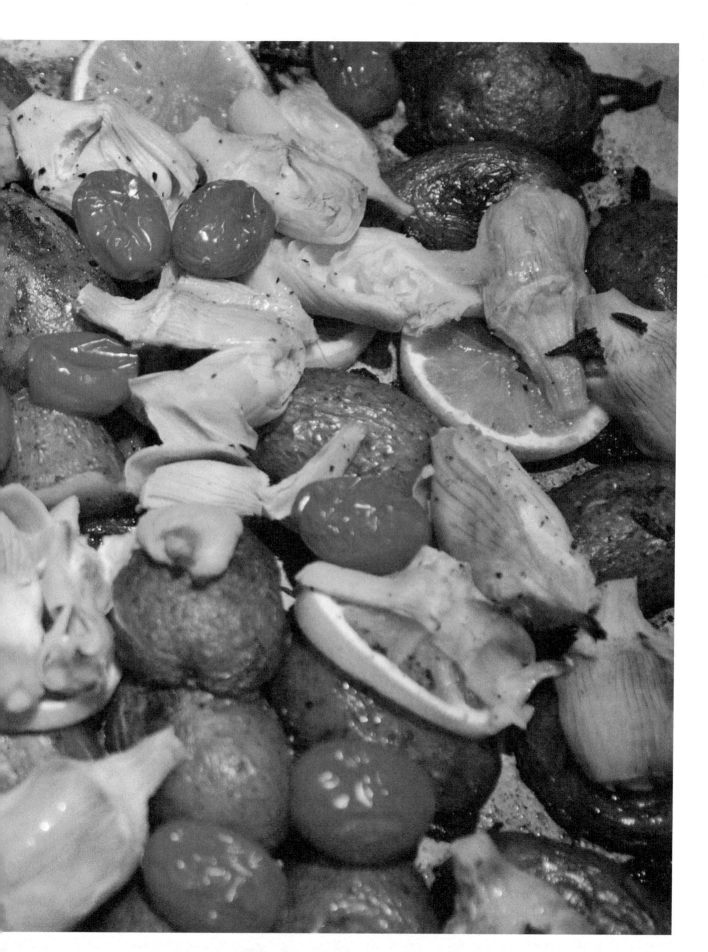

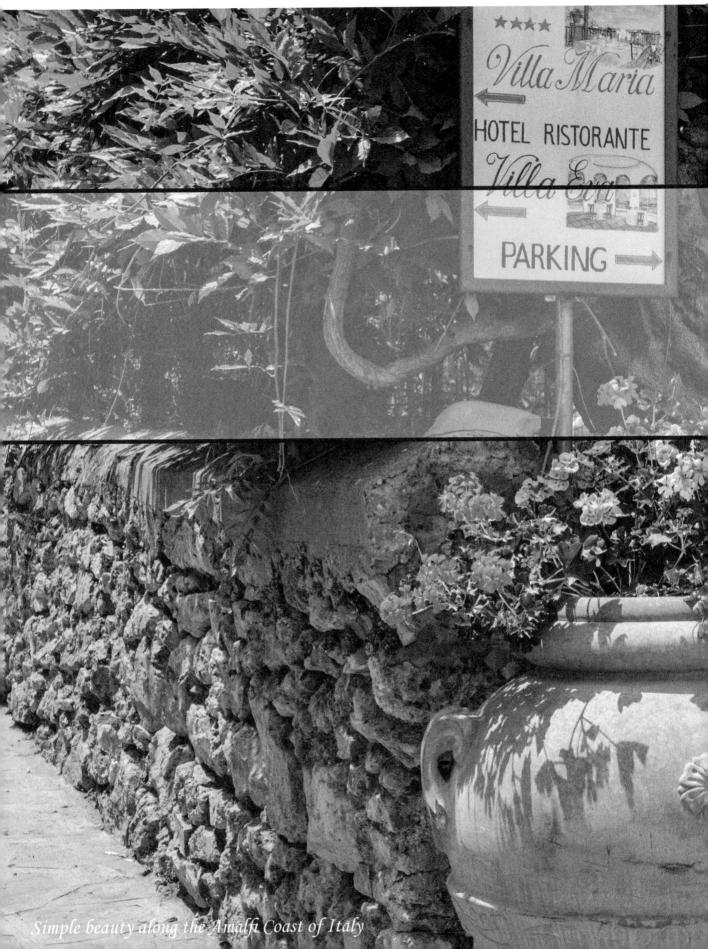

★★★★

Villa Maria

← HOTEL RISTORANTE

Villa Eva

←

PARKING →

Simple beauty along the Amalfi Coast of Italy

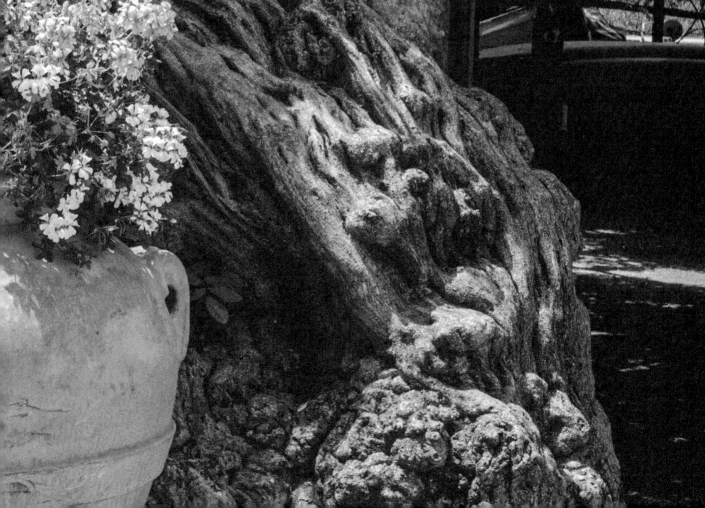

Chapter 7

Desserts

Almond Cranberry Cookies

Almond flour is a great alternative to using wheat flour. You can usually find it in the bulk aisle if your grocer has one. You can make your own almond flour by processing raw almonds in a food processor. However, for these cookies I always purchase almond flour as it's texture is more delicate. It's important not to over bake these. They may not look baked enough when you take them out of the oven but they finish browning when left on the parchment lined baking sheet.

25 minutes prep time
makes 20 cookies

Ingredients

- 2 cups almond flour
- Pinch of salt
- ¼ teaspoon baking soda
- ½ teaspoon ground cinnamon
- 6 tablespoons almond butter
- ¼ cup grade B maple syrup (grade B is darker and is considered the best for baking because it has the most intense flavor but you can use whatever you have)
- 2 teaspoons vanilla
- ½ cup dried cranberries that are sweetened with apple juice
- 2 tablespoons water

Directions

1. Heat the oven to 350 degrees and line a baking sheet with parchment paper.
2. Mix together the almond flour, salt, baking soda and cinnamon in a large mixing bowl.
3. In a medium sized bowl whisk together the almond butter, maple syrup, water and vanilla.
4. Add the wet ingredients to the flour mixture and mix well using a spatula but there is no need to use a mixer. Keep stirring until it all comes together forming a thick dough, then fold in the cranberries.
5. Form dough into balls and place on the prepared baking sheet. The cookies won't spread so no need to allow large spaces between them.
6. Bake for 10 minutes or until the bottoms are browned.
7. Let the cookies cool on the baking sheet for another 5 minutes and transfer to a cooling rack. They will be soft coming out of the oven but will firm up as they cool.

Tip: Cookies will keep 2-3 days in an airtight container but will soften up a bit again when stored

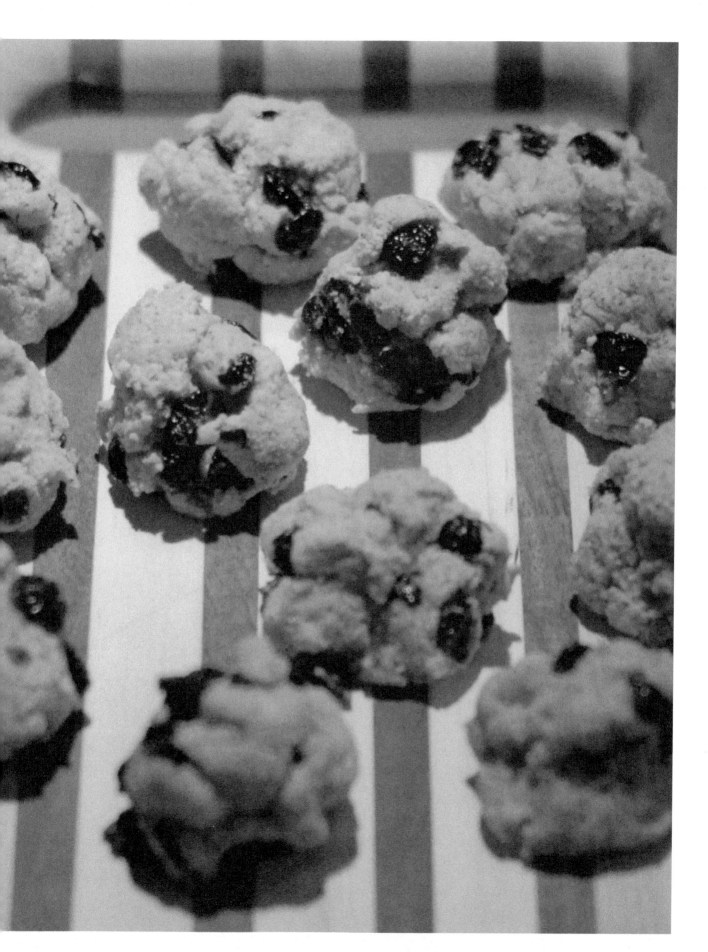

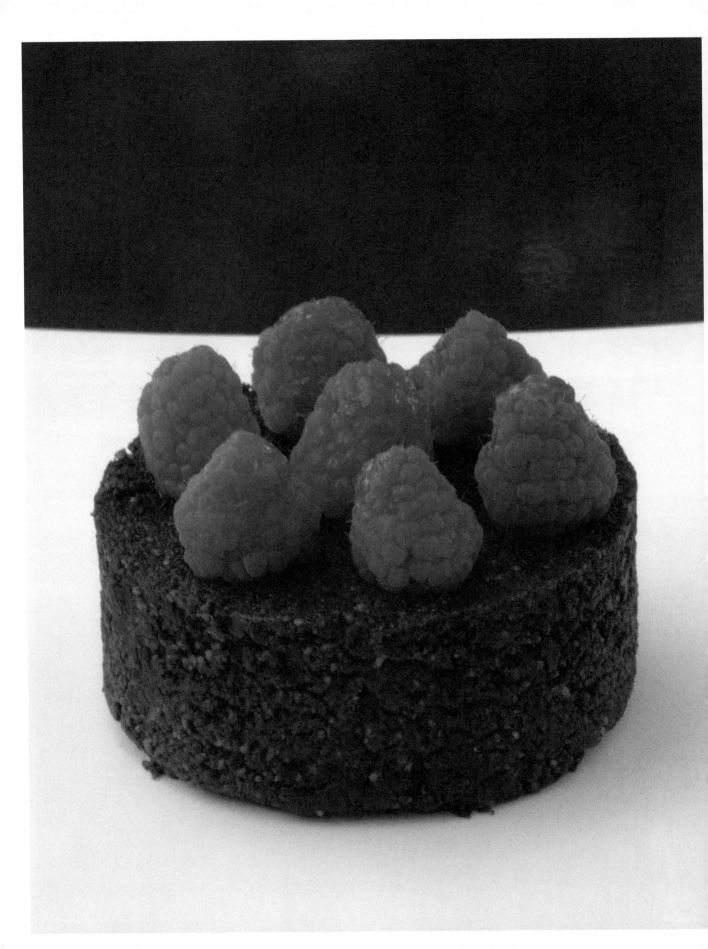

Flourless Chocolate Cake

It's hard to believe this cake is flourless, dairy free, doesn't require baking and yet is so delicious! One "trick" to making these cakes is using a round form so they keep their shape and can easily be cut into slices. They are easy to purchase at most kitchen stores.

10 minutes to make, 2 hours total with chilling time

makes 4 servings

Ingredients

- 1½ cups of raw walnuts
- 8 pitted dates
- ¼ cup raw cacao powder
- ½ teaspoon vanilla extract
- 2 teaspoon water
- Fresh raspberries or other fruit for garnish

Directions

1. Place walnuts in a food processor and process until finely ground.
2. Next add dates, cacao powder and vanilla and process until mixture begins to stick together. Add the water and process briefly. You may or may not use the entire 2 teaspoons of water. Add just enough until the mixture sticks together but doesn't become too sticky.
3. Transfer onto a serving plate and form into a round cake or several smaller bite sized cakes. Chill for approximately 2 hours and decorate with fresh berries. .
4. Take the cake out of the refrigerator one hour before serving.

Almond Jam Dot Cookies

Almond flour is another of my favorite ingredients for baking. I have made my own almond flour by processing oats in the food processor but cookie recipes turn out even by purchasing almond flour in the bulk section of the store. Almond flour is often called almond meal but it's the same product.

25 minutes prep time
makes about 20 cookies

Ingredients

- 1 cup almond flour
- 1½ cup oat flour (use gluten free if you have a sensitivity)
- 2 tablespoons ground flax
- ¼ cup coconut oil, liquefied
- ½ cup maple syrup
- 1 teaspoon vanilla extract
- ½ cup jam – use a brand that is 100% fruit spread with nothing else added

Directions

1. Preheat oven to 350. Line two large baking sheets with parchment paper.
2. Whisk together almond flour, oat flour and flax in a large bowl. In a small bowl stir together coconut oil, maple syrup and vanilla.
3. Add liquid ingredients to dry, and stir until combined.
4. Roll dough into tablespoon-sized balls and arrange them evenly on baking sheets. Flatten the balls and use your thumb to press a 'dot' into the center of each cookie. Fill each well with ½-1 teaspoon of jam.
5. Bake for 12-15 minutes or until golden brown and slightly crispy. Let cool. This cookie will crisp up a bit more upon cooling.

Tip: Although this recipe was originally developed using raspberry jam, using a berry jam seems to work better as it doesn't melt over the cookie while in the oven.

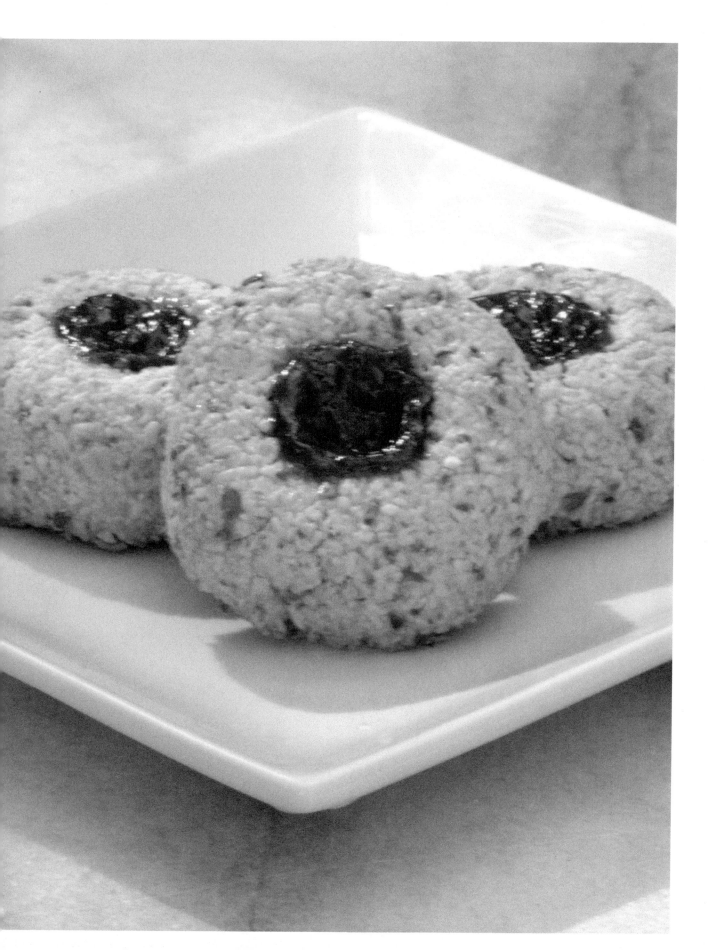

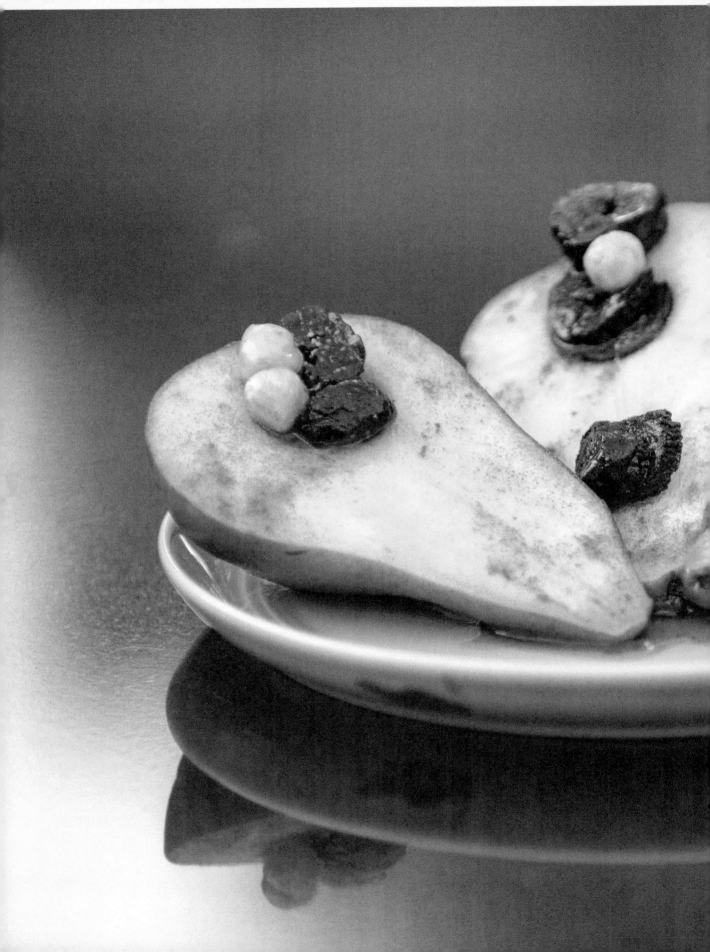

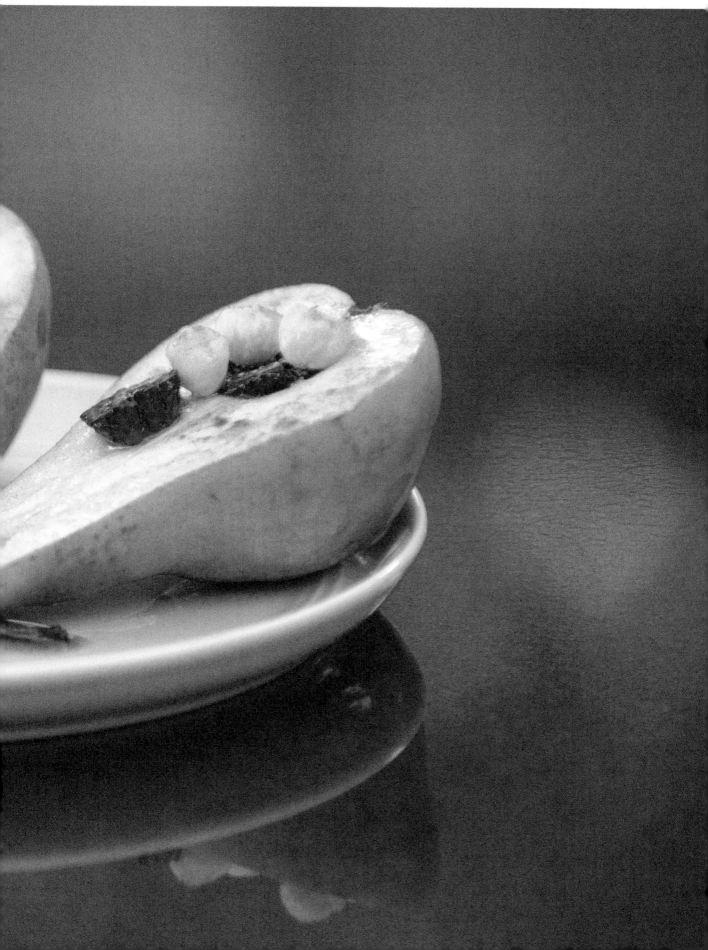

Roasted Pears with Dried Fruit and Hazelnuts

The simplicity and elegance of this dessert is just what's needed at the end of a meal or even leftover as a snack.

30 minutes prep time
makes 4 servings

Ingredients

- 2 ripe Bosc or Bartlett pears (The photo is of a Bosc Pear)
- 4 dried and pitted prunes, chopped in small pieces
- Ground cinnamon, enough to sprinkle tops before roasting
- 4 teaspoons maple syrup – grade B
- 4 teaspoons non-dairy "butter" spread such as Earth Balance
- Small handful of blanched hazelnuts, coarsely chopped or left whole

Directions

1. Preheat the oven to 400 degrees.
2. Cut the pears into halves and using a melon baller or small spoon, carve out the core of the pear halves.
3. Scrape out some of the inside to make enough room for "stuffing" but don't go down too far.
4. Arrange the pears in an ovenproof dish or a glass pie plate.
5. Place the hazelnuts and prunes in the open cavities of the pears, mounding it at the top.
6. Top each pear with a sprinkle of cinnamon, 1 teaspoon non-dairy "butter" and drizzle maple syrup on top.
7. Cover with foil and bake in preheated oven for about 20 minutes, then remove the foil and continue baking until just golden, about 10-15 minutes more. Be sure to check the pears as they are baking. If the juices are sticking to the bottom of the dish you may need to add some water half way through baking.

Moist, Delicious and Gluten Free Apple Cake

This recipe takes a little "doing" but the results are so worth it. It's best served warm right out of the oven. Once you assemble the ingredients and begin it's really pretty easy. Talk about winter comfort food – this is it!

45 minutes prep time
makes 6 generous servings

Ingredients

- ½ cup raw almonds
- ½ cup raw cashews
- 1 small banana
- ½ cup dates, pitted (it's best to buy them fresh with the pits and remove them as you needed, they are fresher that way)
- 2 tablespoons maple syrup
- 1 teaspoon vanilla
- ½ cup coconut oil
- 1 cup oat milk (or homemade almond milk if desired)
- 1 cup plus three tablespoons of all purpose gluten free flour.
- 1 tablespoon baking powder (without aluminum)
- 1 teaspoon baking soda (without aluminum)
- Pinch of salt
- ½ teaspoon cinnamon
- 2-3 crisp, tart apples such as granny smith or honey crisp

Directions

1. Preheat the oven to 350 degrees.
2. Combine the cashews and almonds in a food processor and pulse until you have a fine nut meal that represents coarse flour.
3. Transfer the meal to a separate bowl and add the remaining dry ingredients.
4. Combine the banana, dates, maple syrup, vanilla, coconut oil, and oat milk in the food processor and pulse until you have a smooth mixture.
5. Add the wet mixture to your bowl of dry ingredients, and fold with a rubber scraper. The batter should be thicker than your typical cake batter, but still needs to be moist enough to spread well in a pan. At this point you may need to add a bit of water to achieve a good batter. Just be sure that what you add is no more than 1 teaspoon at a time.
6. Cut up the apples into small cubes and fold them into your batter
7. Spread the batter evenly into a 9" round cake pan. Bake for 25 to 35 minutes or until firm to the touch.
8. An optional finish for the cake could be homemade applesauce as a "frosting" which is a wonderful addition.

Note: To make 1 cup of homemade applesauce with fresh apples start by dicing (leave skin on) and roasting them in a pan at 400 degrees for about one hour until soft. Sprinkle with cinnamon before roasting. When apples are finished roasting, process in food processor until smooth. You can completely eliminate this step if you wish and top the cake with dried cranberries and nuts instead, however the warm fresh applesauce is wonderful. For the flour component Whole Foods sells a combination of garbanzo and fava bean flour with potato starch in it. It makes a delicious cake. I've also used half of the all purpose gluten free flour and half coconut flour in this recipe and it gives a nutty, heavier texture that is also delicious. This recipe is heavily adapted from Veg with an Edge recipes.

Panna Cotta with Blackberry Sauce

"Panna Cotta" means cooked cream and it's usually a dairy and gelatin based dessert. The use of non- dairy milk and agar and arrowroot for thickeners is uniquely delicious and light.

25 minutes prep time
makes 4 servings

Ingredients

Panna Cotta:
- 2 cups unsweetened coconut milk
- 1½ cups cashew milk
- ¼ cup pure maple syrup, grade B if you can find it
- 1½ tablespoons agar flakes
- 2 teaspoons vanilla

Blackberry Sauce:
- 1 cup fresh blackberries
- 2 tablespoons date sugar
- Zest of one lemon
- ¼ cup water
- Juice from one lemon
- 1 tablespoon arrowroot flour

Directions

1. Place the coconut milk, cashew milk and maple syrup in Vita Mix and blend on low speed until combined.
2. Remove one cup of this mixture and heat it in a small saucepan. Add the agar flakes and stir together for about 3 minutes. The agar flakes will not completely dissolve. This is normal and doesn't affect the outcome of the recipe.
3. Put the rest of the mixture in a large pan. Bring to a boil and reduce to a simmer.
4. Add the agar mixture and stir gently for about 10 minutes. Add vanilla the last few minutes of cooking.
5. Cool slightly and pour into individual dishes. Put in the refrigerator and allow the panna cotta to set up for at least a couple of hours. Once the panna cotta is completely set up, top with blackberry sauce.
6. For the blackberry sauce start by stirring together the blackberries, date sugar, lemon zest and water in a small saucepan. Press lightly on the blackberries to release some of the juices. Cook on medium to low heat until the blackberries are softened which usually takes between 5-7 minutes. Stir occasionally.
7. In a small bowl, stir together the lemon juice and arrowroot until the mixture becomes creamy looking. Pour this mixture over the blackberries in the pan and cook together for another 2 minutes or until a thick sauce comes together.
8. Let the sauce cool and use it to top the panna cotta right before serving.

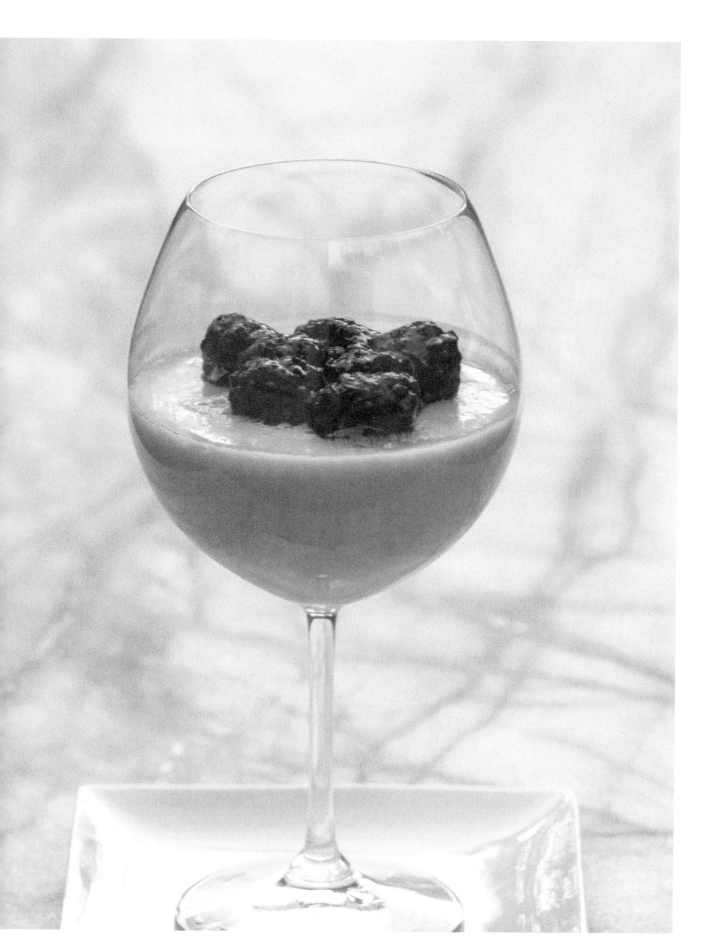

Berries and Balsamic Dessert

This is probably the simplest dessert you will ever make and yet it is satisfying and an elegant finish to any dinner. What a great way to get your serving of fruit!

5 minutes prep time
makes 4 servings

Ingredients

- 3 cups of fresh or frozen berries (a mixture of raspberries, blueberries, strawberries and/or blackberries)
- Bordeaux chocolate, Fig or Cocoa Crema balsamic vinegar to taste

Directions

1. Place ¾ cup of berries in each of four bowls. Drizzle to taste with your choice of balsamic vinegar. Enjoy!

Tip: In the winter I purchase bags of frozen berries to use when fresh are unavailable. The taste is wonderful and sometimes frozen fruit (without added sugar or preservative) is as fresh as fruit from the summer because it is picked and quick frozen at its peak.

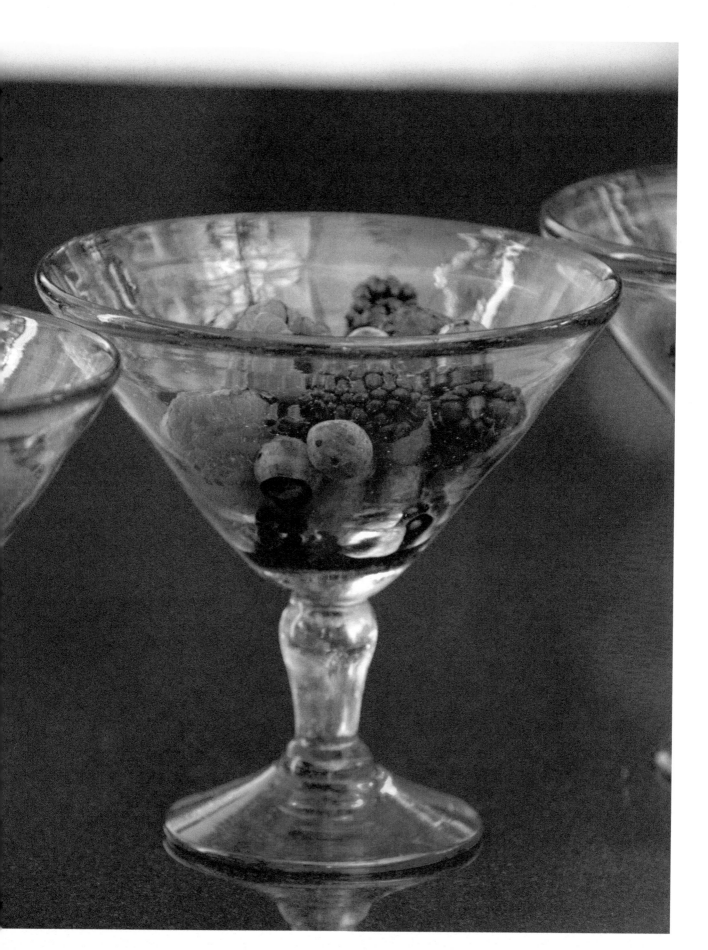

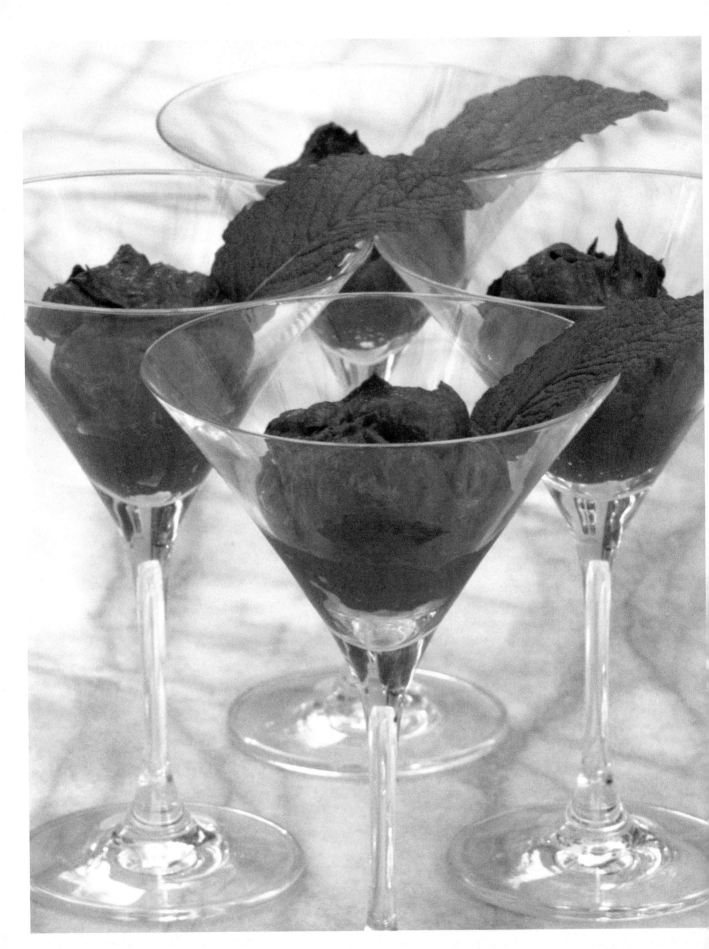

Quick, Delicious and Healthful Chocolate Pudding

Many times avocados provide the creamy texture and taste in that's needed in recipes, especially when they are at the peak of ripeness. If using for dinner guests (or is you just want to spoil yourself or a friend) serve it up in elegant presentation by putting it in pretty glass dishes and top with a sprig of mint for garnish.

5 minutes prep time and 2 hours in the refrigerator
makes4 servings

Ingredients

- 2 ripe (not overly ripe) bananas
- 2 ripe avocados (should be ripe enough to be soft to the touch and maybe a little dark in color on the outside)
- 6-8 tablespoons of raw cacao (if difficult to find use the best organic ground cocoa that you can find)
- 1 teaspoon vanilla extract or scrape the inside of one small vanilla bean
- 1 teaspoon of cinnamon

Directions

1. Process the avocados and banana in a food processor until smooth. You may need to stop once in a while to scrape down the mixture once or twice while processing.
2. Add the vanilla, cacao and cinnamon and process until blended.
3. Refrigerate for at least two hours to allow it to set up before serving.

Blueberry Cashew Cream Cheesecake

It took me a while to try using cashews for achieving a creamy base similar to cream cheese. As with all nuts, cashews are very calorie dense. While I'm not a "calorie counter" two cups of nuts can really add up. The flip side however is the lovely dessert that emerges right before your eyes for those special dinners or when you are bringing a wonderfully unique hostess gift.

30 minutes prep time and 3-4 hours soaking time for the cashews
makes 4 servings

Ingredients

Crust:
- 1 cup pecans
- ¾ cup medjool dates, pits removed

Filling:
- 2 cups raw cashews, soaked (cover with cool water for 3-4 hours)
- 4 tablespoons lemon juice
- ¾ cup fresh blueberries
- 2 teaspoon vanilla
- 1 tablespoon psyllium husk (this is used as a binder to set the cheesecake)
- ⅓ cup date sugar

Directions

1. Pulse the dates and pecans in a food processor. Process until you have a "paste like" consistency and pecans are finely chopped.
2. Press the pecan and date mixture into the bottom of an 8" round pan lined with parchment paper. Wash the bowl of the food processor and dry well.
3. Pour off the soaking water from the cashews, rinse them well and drain.
4. Add the lemon juice, vanilla, date sugar, cashews and psyllium husk in the order just given.
5. Process in the food processor until you have a creamy textured mixture which takes about 3-5 minutes.
6. Add the blueberries and process again. You will most likely need to stop the processing at regular intervals and use a spatula to clean the sides.
7. You will want a thick and creamy filling but not dry. If it appears too dry you may add a tablespoon of water at time.
8. Once you have processed your "cashew cream" pour it onto the crust and spread evenly.
9. Refrigerate at least one hour before serving.

Tip: If you do not have an 8" round pan you may use a 9" springform pan but the cheesecake will not be as high.

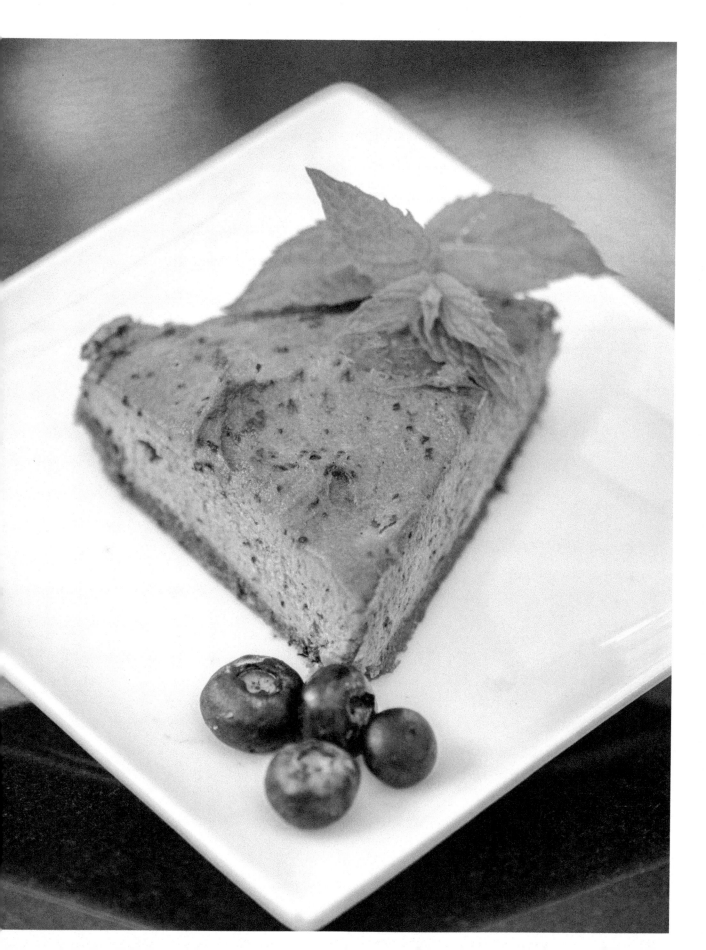

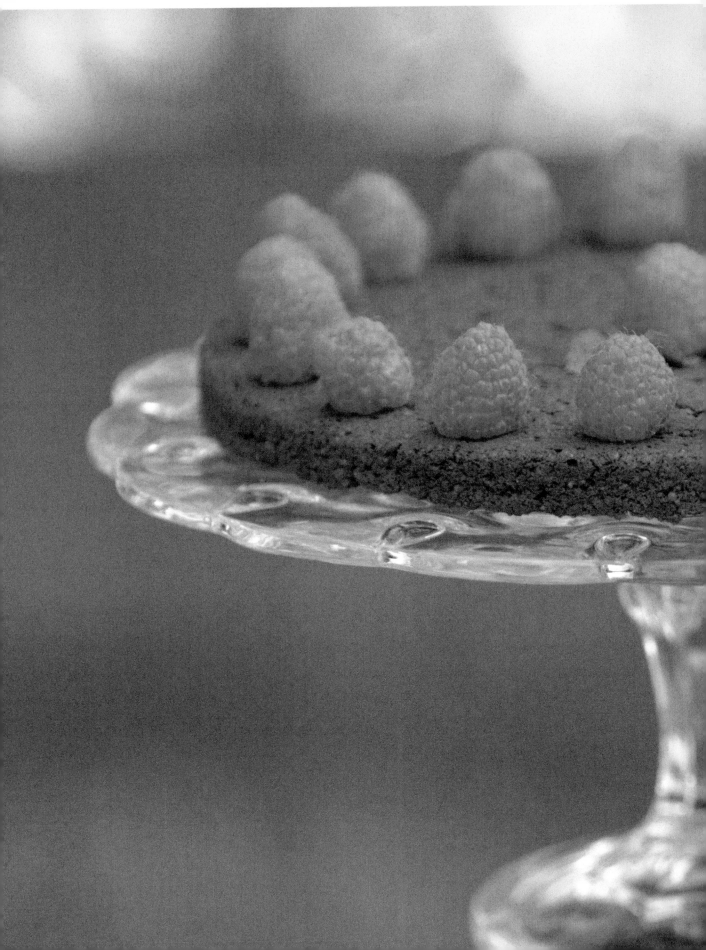

Elegant, Delicious and Healthful Chocolate Cake

This simple cake is elegant when topped with berries and sliced thinly. If you prefer a higher cake double the recipe and make two layers.

30 minutes prep time
makes 6 servings

Ingredients

- 1½ cups oat flour
- ⅓ cup unsweetened cocoa
- 1 teaspoon baking soda
- 1 cup date sugar
- Pinch of salt
- 3 tablespoons coconut oil, liquefied
- 1 cup cold water
- 1½ teaspoon vanilla
- 1 tablespoon apple cider vinegar (Braggs Apple Cider Vinegar if available)
- About 5 large strawberries or a pint of raspberries for topping

Directions

1. Heat the oven to 350 degrees.
2. Mix together the oat flour, cocoa, baking soda, pinch of salt and date sugar.
3. In a separate bowl whisk together the water, oil, vanilla and apple cider vinegar.
4. Add the liquid mixture to dry ingredients and mix well. You can do this by hand or with and electric mixer. Using a mixer will make the cake rise a bit more.
5. Place the mixture in a non-stick 9" round baking pan - preferably a heavy pan that holds the heat.
6. Bake for 20 minutes or until the top springs back when pressed gently or when a toothpick comes out clean.

Tip: You can easily make your own oat flour with a food processor by processing 1½ cups of rolled oats until they are of "flour-like" consistency. It will still have some texture to it and that's OK.

Oatmeal Berry Cobbler

I call this a winter comfort food. When berries are out of season the next best option is using organically grown frozen berries. The oatmeal, berries and other flavors combine for a warm dessert or snack that is quick to make.

10 minutes prep time
makes 2 servings

Ingredients

- 1⅓ cup frozen mixed berries (organic if possible)
- ⅔ cup oatmeal
- ¾ cup water
- 2 tablespoons raisins (large golden raisins work well if you can find them)
- ⅛ teaspoon vanilla
- 2 tablespoons chopped raw walnuts
- ¼ teaspoon cinnamon

Directions

1. Combine the berries, oats, raisins and vanilla in a small saucepan.
2. Add the water (you may need to adjust to more or less water depending on the consistency you like).
3. Cook on medium high heat until bubbling. Add walnuts and cinnamon. Cook another 5 minutes stirring occasionally and adding additional water if needed.
4. Serve warm and enjoy!

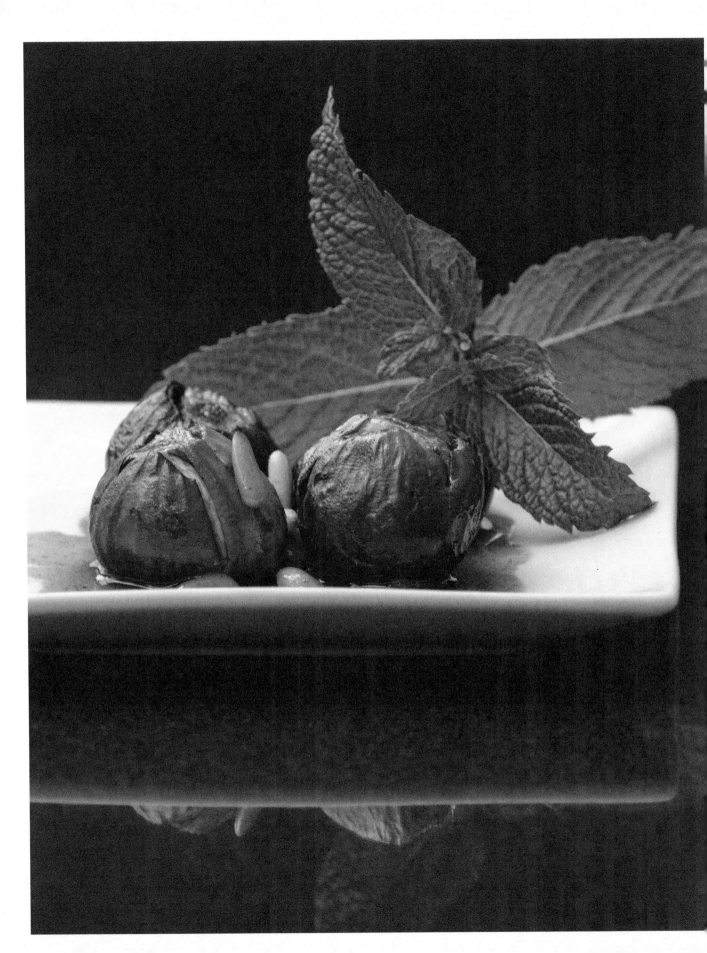

Oven Roasted Figs and Pine Nuts

Figs are low in calories. However, they contain health benefiting soluble dietary fiber, minerals, vitamins, and pigment anti-oxidants that contribute immensely towards optimum health and wellness. Roasting them intensifies the flavor!

25 minutes prep time including roasting
makes 2 servings

Ingredients

- Four fresh figs
- Port or Madeira wine to cover the bottom of the roasting pan
- 2 tablespoons pine nuts
- Sprinkle of date or brown sugar

Directions

1. Preheat the oven at 350 degrees
2. Cut the stalks off the figs and cut a cross in the top about ⅓ of the way through.
3. Stand them in an oven-proof baking dish and pour enough wine over them and cover the bottom of the baking dish. You don't need a lot of wine but enough to have basted the figs with wine and to lightly cover the bottom of the pan.
4. Scatter the pine nuts over the figs and sprinkle with the sugar.
5. Bake in the preheated oven for about 20 minutes. Check on them occasionally to make sure they aren't drying out in the oven and baste as needed.

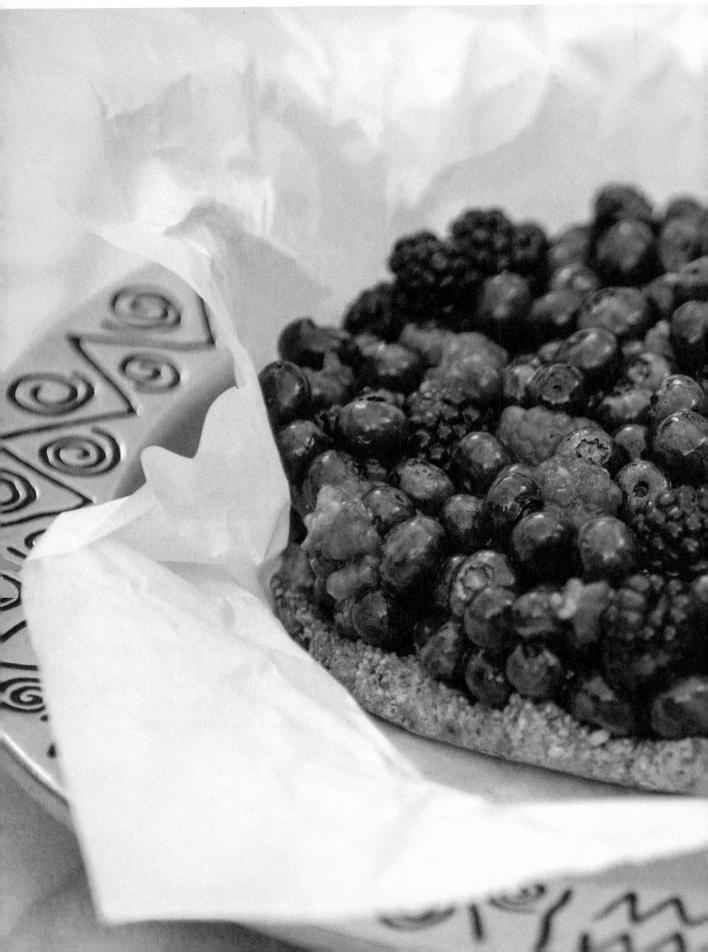

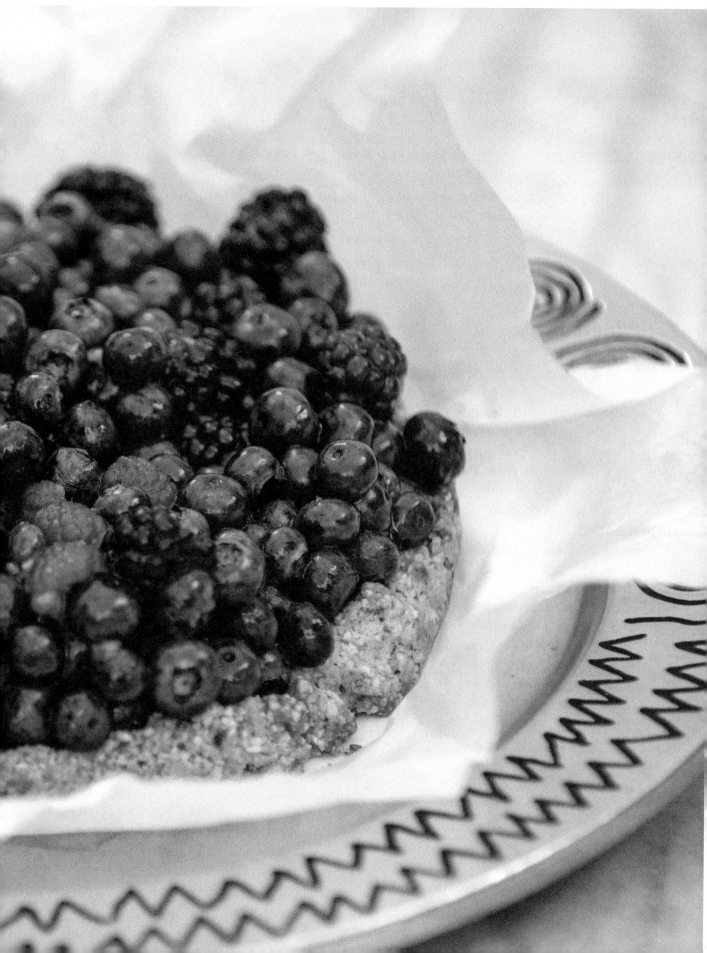

Berry Tart with Toasted Almond Crust

I enjoy entertaining guests and I always love to surprise them with a beautiful and delicious plant based dessert that "wows" at the end of the meal. This one does it!

25 minutes prep time and 1 hour cooling time
makes 12 small servings

Ingredients

Crust:
- 2 tablespoons coconut oil, liquefied
- ⅔ cup toasted almonds
- ¼ cup oats
- ⅔ cup garbanzo bean flour
- 3 tablespoons maple syrup (grade B if possible)
- 1 teaspoon vanilla

Filling:
- 1¾ pints of blueberries
- 1 pint raspberries
- ½ pint blackberries
- 2 tablespoons maple syrup (grade B if possible)
- ¾ cup apple juice, reserve one tablespoon aside
- ¾ teaspoon agar flakes
- 1 teaspoon arrowroot
- ½ teaspoon vanilla

Directions

1. Preheat the oven to 350 degrees and line a 9" spring form pan with parchment paper.
2. Place the almonds and oats in food processor and process until finely ground.
3. Transfer almonds and oats to a bowl and add the rest of the ingredients for the crust. Mix together until you have evenly moistened dough.
4. Press the dough onto the bottom and sides (about half way up the sides) of the spring form pan. Bake for 18-20 minutes until golden brown.
5. Remove from the oven and let cool.
6. To make the filling combine the apple juice (remember to reserve 1 tablespoon) and agar flakes in a small heavy bottom pan. Bring to a boil, whisk together and reduce the heat. Let the mixture simmer for about 5 minutes or until the agar flakes are completely dissolved. Stir occasionally while simmering.
7. In a small bowl mix together the tablespoon of apple juice with the teaspoon of arrowroot. Add this to the small pan of apple juice and agar and whisk together until the mixture thickens. Once thick, remove from the heat and add the maple syrup and vanilla. Let this mixture cool slightly and thicken a little more upon cooling.
8. Combine the berries in a large bowl, mix with the cooled liquid above and place in the crust. Refrigerate for at least an hour allowing the filling to set. The tart will keep overnight if needed but the crust does become a little soggy if it sits too long.

Chocolate Pecan Cookies

Nut flours such as almond and bean flour (garbanzo bean) adds taste, texture and nutrition to recipes. I haven't used wheat flour in baking for so long I don't even think about it. A word of caution; remember that any flour is highly processed and is low in fiber. Recipes like this are great but are special treats.

20 minutes prep time
makes about a dozen cookies depending on the size

Ingredients

- 2 large apples, diced with skin on
- 2 teaspoon vanilla
- 1 cup chopped pitted dates
- 1 cup garbanzo bean flour
- 4 tablespoons raw cacao
- ¾ cup oats
- ¾ cup pecans, chopped

Directions

1. Preheat the oven to 350 degrees.
2. Place the apples, vanilla and dates in the food processor and process until you have blended everything together and it is creamy. You will probably have to stop at one or two intervals and use a spatula to move the mixture back down into the processor bowl.
3. In another bowl whisk together the dry ingredients (except pecans) until well blended.
4. Add the creamy mixture from the food processor and mix well. Add the pecans at the very end.
5. Bake on a parchment paper lined baking sheet for about 10 minutes.
6. The bottom of the cookie browns quickly so watch them when you are getting close to 10 minutes in the oven.
7. Cool on rack and enjoy!

Tip: Medjool dates are best if you can find them, purchase them with pits and remove the pits right before using – they are much fresher this way. If you don't have raw cacao available you can always substitute ground cacao.

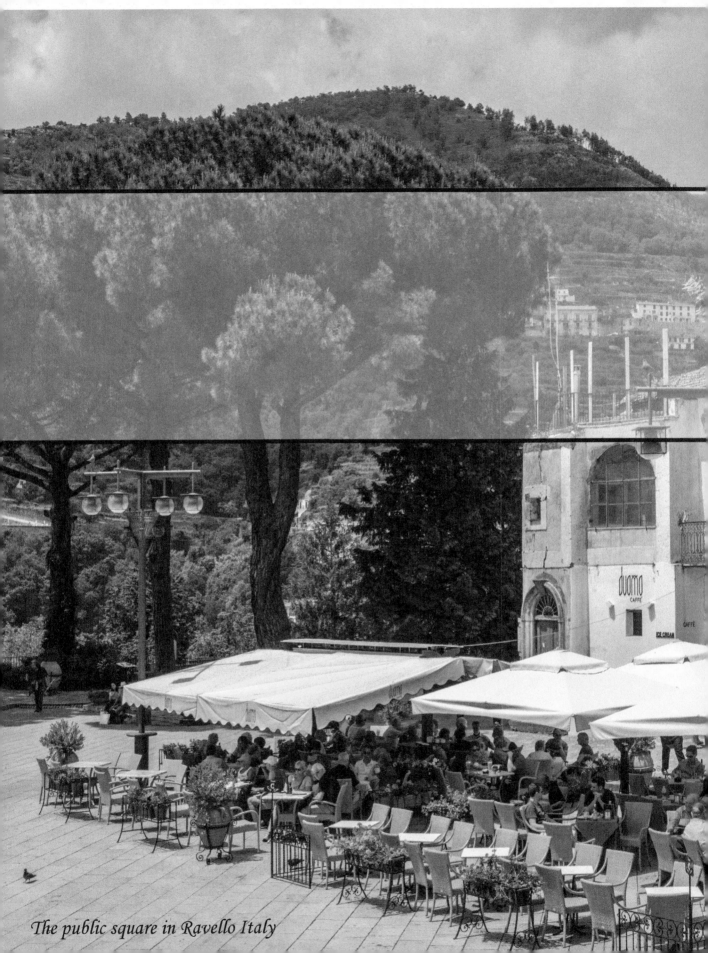

The public square in Ravello Italy

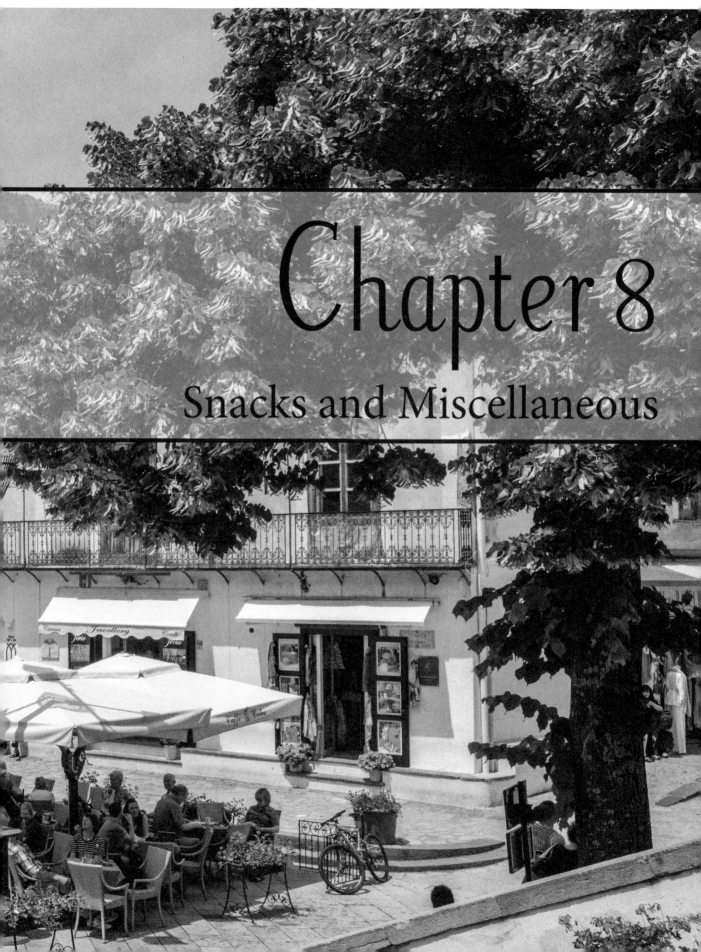

Chapter 8
Snacks and Miscellaneous

High Protein, No Nut Chocolate Dessert or Snack

This easy to make snack or dessert is perfect for people who have nut allergies and yet it's a wonderful snack for anyone that keeps well in the freezer. They are loaded with fiber, antioxidants and flavor.

10 minutes prep time
makes 12 servings

Ingredients

- 1 cup dates
- ¼ cup hulled hemp seeds
- ¼ cup chia seeds
- ¼ cup sesame seeds
- ¼ cup of raw cacao (you can substitute ground cocoa if needed)
- ½ teaspoon vanilla extract or you can use Fiori d'Sicilia to add a citrus flavor
- ¼ teaspoon cinnamon
- ¼ cup raw cacao nibs
- ½ cup dried cranberries

Directions

1. Process the pitted dates in a food processor until they form a chunky paste.
2. Add all other ingredients, except for the cacao nibs, and pulse until combined. Stop as needed to push the mixture down into the food processor bowl to make sure everything is mixed well.
3. Add the cacao nibs and pulse together.
4. You should have dough that is sticky enough to form into balls. If the dough is not sticky enough you may need to add a tablespoon of water at a time to make it stickier to form a ball. Be careful not to add too much water or your dough will be too thin.
5. Shape into small balls and freeze for at least 20 minutes for them to set before serving.

Tip: Buy dates with the pits in as they are fresher and remove the pits just before using. You can find Fiori d'Sicilia online through King Arthur flour. I have also found that the consistency of the dough usually depends on the freshness of the dates. Very fresh dates will be creamy and moist. If you happen to purchase an older inventory of dates at the store the dough will be drier. A good way to tell is to squeeze the box to test how firm (older) or soft (fresher) the dates are.

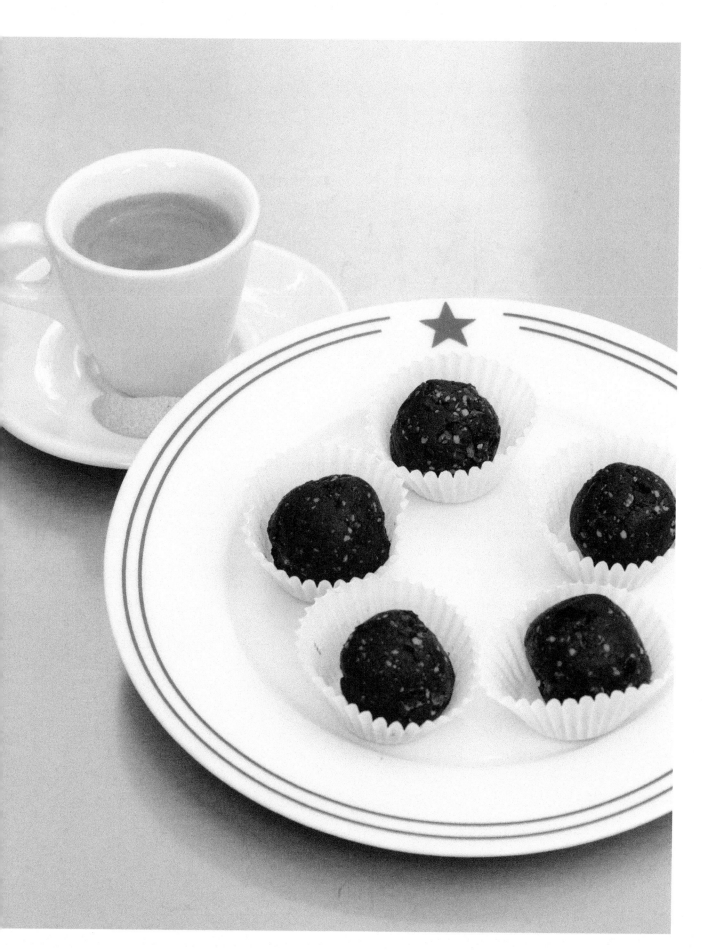

Gremolata

This garnish can be used over quinoa or as a side dish on its own. Its mixture of sweet, sour, bitter and fresh adds an amazing flavor "sensation" wherever it is used.

10 minutes prep time
served as a garnish

Ingredients

- Six scallions as fresh as you can find them
- 2 small lemons preferably Meyer lemons if you can find them
- 2-3 garlic cloves with skins on
- Small handful of fresh parsley, chopped finely

Directions

1. Preheat a hot grill surface.
2. Cut off the roots of the scallions and chop within an inch of the tops of the greens. Cut the lemons into thin slices but leave the skins on
3. Toss the scallions, lemons and garlic together and grill until the scallions are charred and the garlic softens. Do not let the garlic get brown. Add salt and pepper if desired.
4. Remove from heat, peel the garlic and chop finely once its cooled.
5. Mix the garlic together with other ingredients and enjoy!

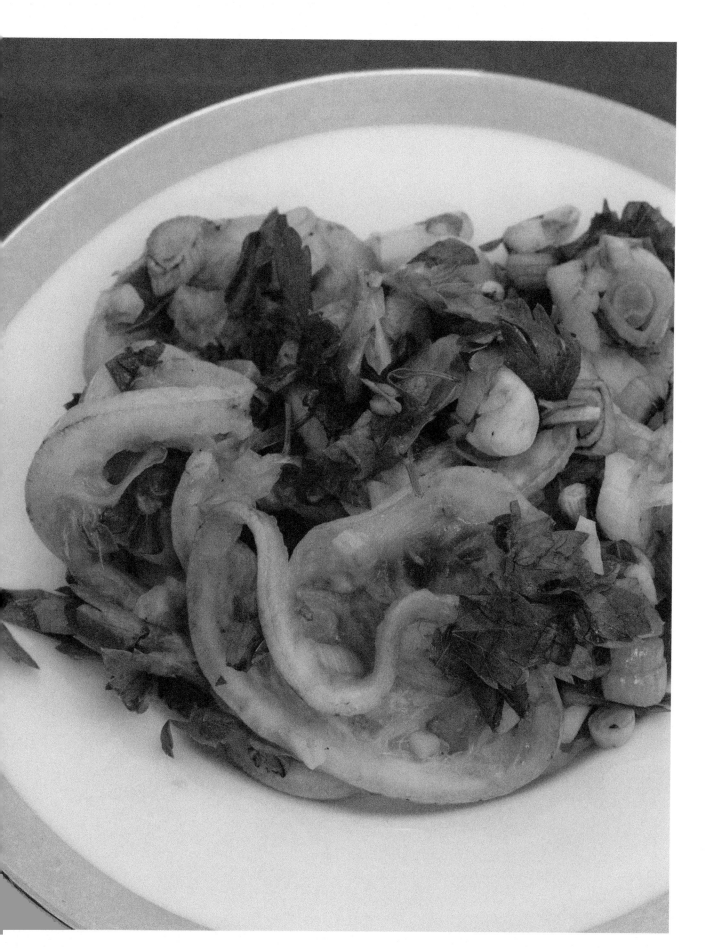

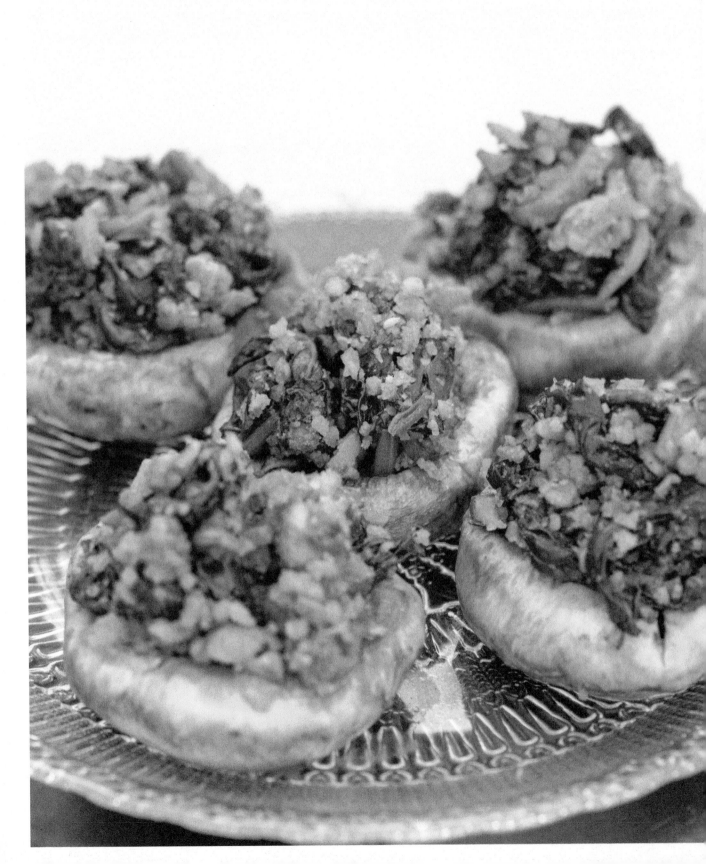

Stuffed Mushrooms with Spinach and Walnuts

These are delicious and easy to make. They can be arranged on a platter as an appetizer or placed on small plates in groups of three to serve as a first course for a sit down dinner.

10 minutes prep time
makes about 12 mushrooms depending on the mushroom size

Ingredients

- 1 pound white mushrooms, wiped clean with a paper towel
- 3 cloves of roasted garlic, roasted in their skins
- 2 teaspoons olive oil (optional)
- 1 pound lightly steamed spinach
- 1 cup fresh walnuts, chopped finely in a food processor
- Freshly ground black pepper

Directions

1. Preheat the oven to 400 degrees. Line a heavy baking pan with parchment paper.
2. Remove the stems from the mushrooms but reserve them for the stuffing.
3. Place the mushroom caps on the parchment paper and bake for about 7 minutes or until the bottoms of mushrooms are browned.
4. Chop the mushroom stems and place them in a skillet with the roasted garlic. Cook them together for about 3 minutes and add the optional oil.
5. Stir in the spinach, walnuts and fresh ground pepper.
6. Fill the mushroom caps with the filling mixture and arrange in the baking pan with lined parchment paper. Bake 10 minutes until mushrooms are tender and filling is hot.

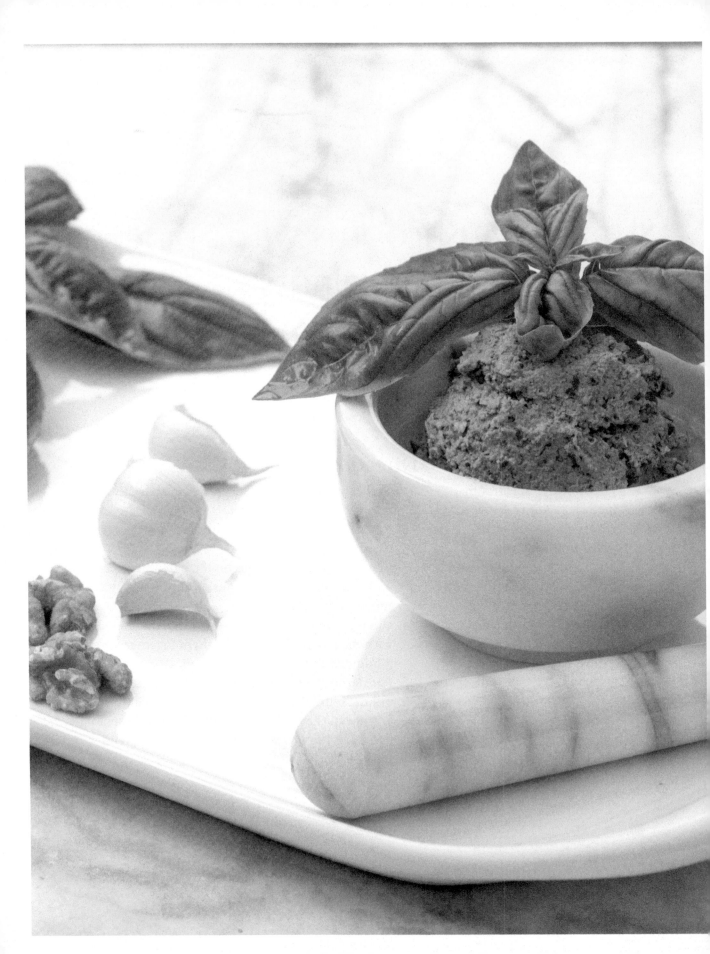

Basil Walnut Pesto

If you love pesto but want to avoid the calories and saturated fat in olive oil or the fat in cheese, this recipe is for you. The cannelloni beans are a creamy substitute for oil and the nutritional yeast adds a cheesy flavor along with vitamin B-12.

10 minutes prep time
makes 1 cup

Ingredients

- A medium sized bunch of fresh basil
- 2-3 cloves of garlic depending on your taste
- 1 cup raw walnuts
- 1 tablespoon water
- ½ cup cannelloni beans
- 1 tablespoon nutritional yeast
- Salt, pepper to taste
- Juice of ½ lemon
- Additional 1-2 tablespoons water, if needed, to add at the end for consistency

Directions

1. Place the basil, garlic, tablespoon of water and walnuts in a food processor and process until finely blended. You may have to use a spatula to press down the mixture a couple of times.
2. Add the beans, nutritional yeast, salt, pepper and lemon juice and process together until smooth. Add water if needed and salt and pepper again if needed to taste.

Walnut Sage Pesto

Combining the flavors of walnuts and sage with the creaminess of the cannelloni beans makes this a great tasting and nutrient dense pesto.

10 minutes prep time
makes about 1 cup

Ingredients

- ¼ cup fresh sage
- ¼ cup cannelloni beans
- 3 cloves of garlic, crushed
- ⅓ cup roasted walnuts

Directions

1. Place the roasted walnuts in a food processor and process. Add rest of ingredients and pulse until combined.

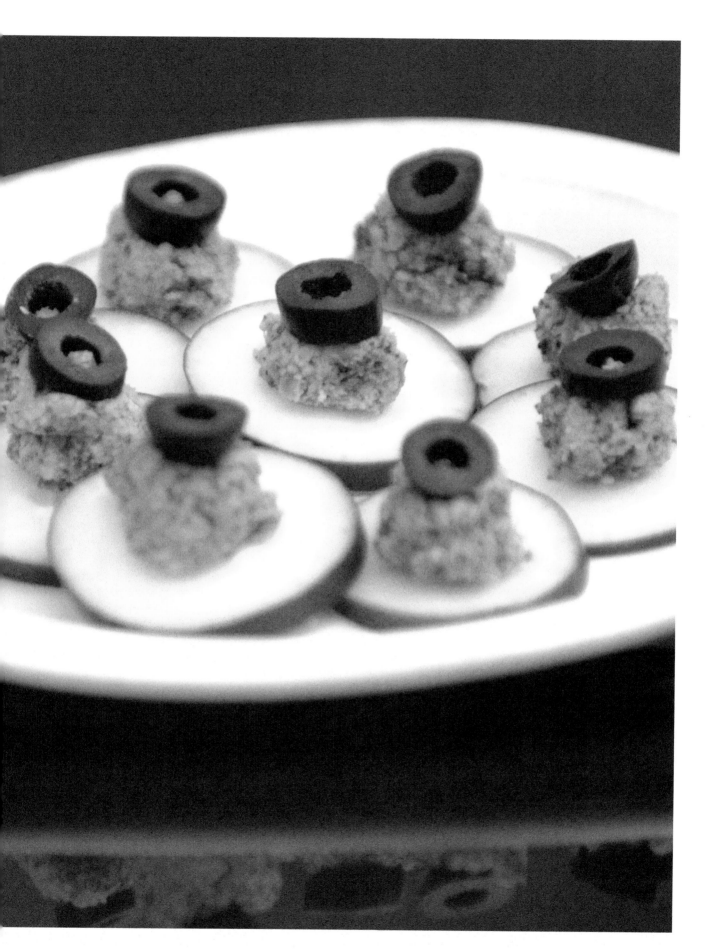

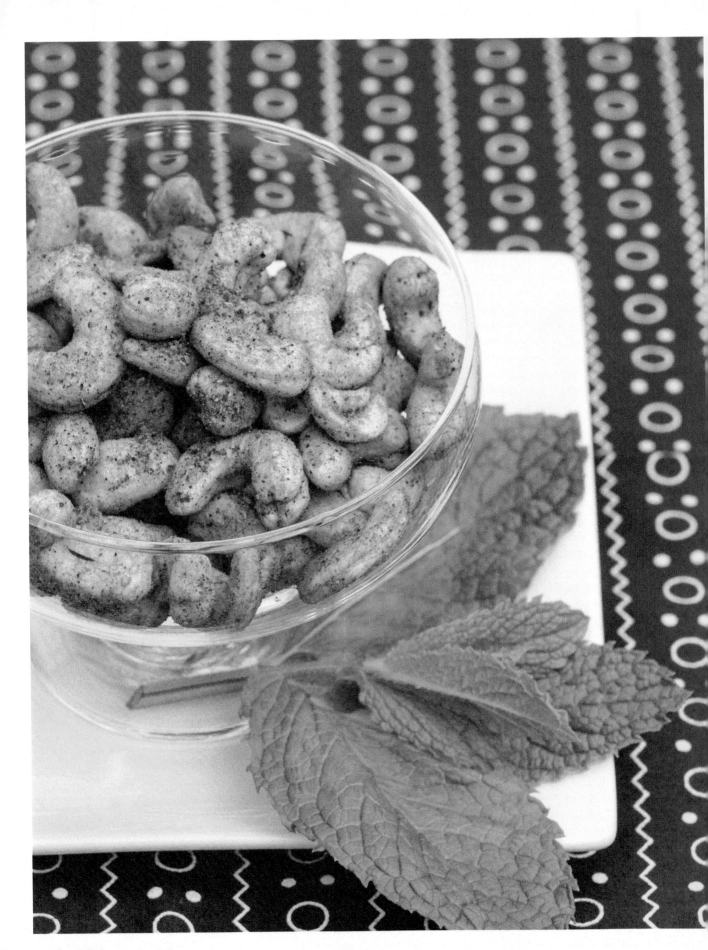

Hot and Spicy Turmeric Cashews

This quick and easy recipe is a great way to add the powerful antioxidant turmeric to your diet. I love to have a small bowl of these out at dinner parties and guests always enjoy them.

12 minutes prep time
makes 1 cup

Ingredients

- 1 cup raw cashews
- scant sesame oil
- ¼ teaspoon fine grain sea salt or to taste
- 1½ teaspoons sesame seeds
- ½ teaspoon cayenne pepper or hot chili powder
- ½ tablespoon ground turmeric

Directions

1. Spray the cashews with a scant amount of sesame oil, just enough so the spices stick to the cashews. Add sea salt, sesame seeds, cayenne pepper or chili powder and turmeric.
2. Taste and adjust the seasonings per your preference.

Blooming Onion

*Here's a great way to get the antioxidant benefits from eating a whole onion.
It's not hard to do when presented like this. The blooming onion can easily be
served as an appetizer or as a side with dinner.*

about an hour but most the time is for baking
number of servings depend on whether you use it as a side or appetizer

Ingredients

- 1 large onion (Vidalia if available)
- ¼ cup gluten free Panko style breadcrumbs
- 1 tablespoon, or to taste, red chili or cayenne pepper
- 2 tablespoon ground flax
- 6 tablespoon water

Directions

1. Heat the oven to 400 degrees.
2. Combine the ground flax and water and let stand for about 10 minutes or until it develops the consistency of an egg.
3. Cut the top of the onion (not the root end but the top) about ½ inch down from the top. Remove the outermost layers of the onion. Rest the onion on its side or on the cut end and cut the onion into about 16 sections. The actual number of sections may vary depending on the size of the onion. Make sure the sections are no wider than ½ inch. Peel the sections down to the root but leave the root intact.
4. Place the onion on a baking sheet or baking plate (I used a pie plate) and pull the sections open. If some of the sections are not opening easily you may have to slice them a little further to open.
5. Mix together the breadcrumbs, spice and egg in a small bowl.
6. Open each section and place the "stuffing" mixture inside each one.
7. Cover the onion with foil and bake for 10 minutes. This begins the cooking process and steams everything together. After 10 minutes remove the cover and bake another 35-40 minutes or until the tops of the onion are browned and the "petals" are cooked through.

Tip: If you want a more simplified version of this recipe it will also
work with just using the gluten free breadcrumbs, spice and water as
the "filling."

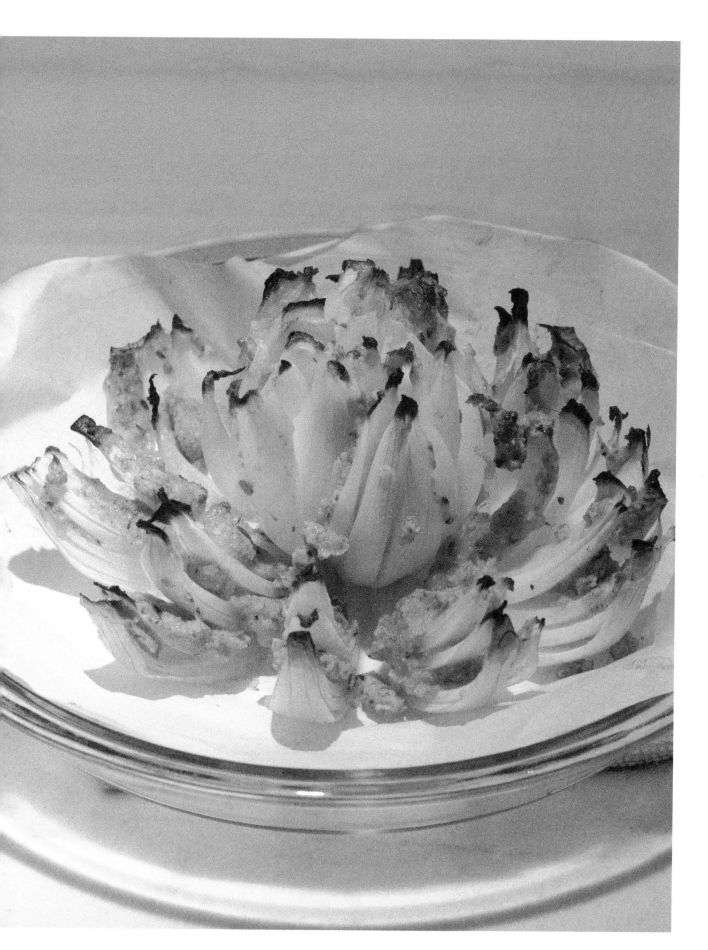

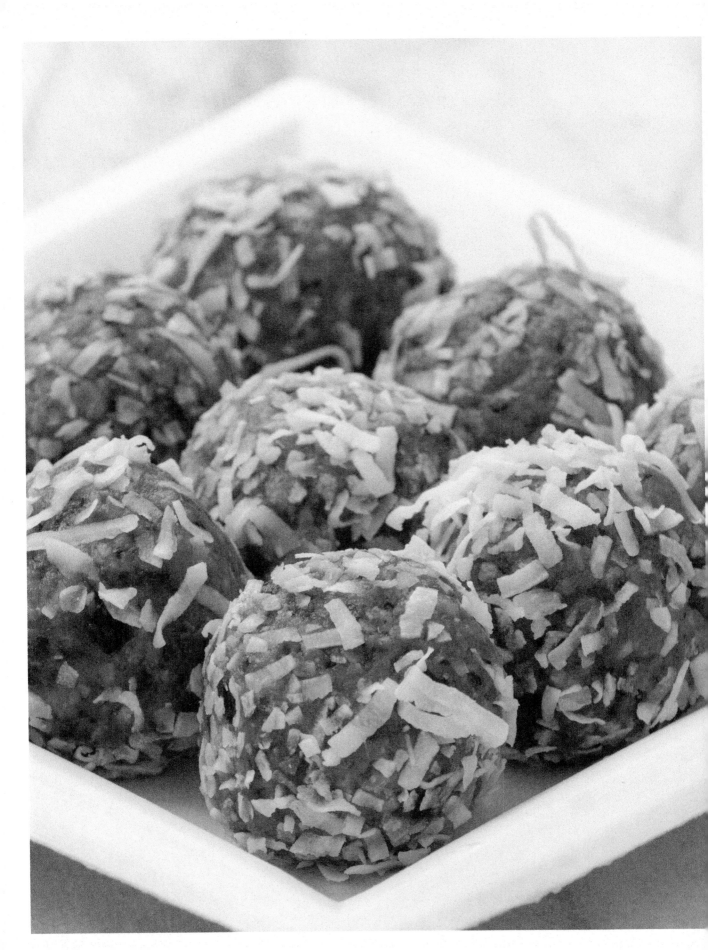

Almond, Cranberry and Orange Energy Snack

This is a quick and easy snack or dessert. I like having foods like this available in my refrigerator or freezer when needed for company or to bring for a pot luck dinner. You may want to do some adjusting if the mixture is too moist or dry. If too moist add more coconut and if too dry add an additional teaspoon of the maple syrup.

5 minutes prep time
makes about 15 snacks

Ingredients

- 1 cup unsweetened finely shredded coconut
- 1 cup almond butter
- 1 cup dried cranberries
- ¼ cup grade B maple syrup
- Zest of one organically grown orange.

Directions

1. Measure out ½ cup of the shredded coconut.
2. Place the ½ cup of coconut and rest of ingredients in a food processor and mix well.
3. Roll into bite size balls.
4. Roll the finished balls in the other half of the coconut.
5. These store well in the freezer or can be kept in the refrigerator is using immediately.

Tip: If you can't find an organic orange be sure to double, even triple, wash the orange.

Chia Seed Jam

When fresh berries are in season it's a wonderful time to make jam. After "trial and error" I found a way make this fresh tasting and healthful jam to have on hand. Chia seeds are a natural thickener and they add additional fiber that lowers the glycemic index of the berries which is already lower than most other fruit. If you want to avoid any sweetener at all you can eliminate the maple syrup in the recipe entirely

15 minutes prep time
makes 1 cup

Ingredients

- 3 cups fresh or frozen organic raspberries, blackberries, blueberries or strawberries
- 3 to 4 tablespoons pure maple syrup
- 2 tablespoons chia seeds
- 1 teaspoon pure vanilla extract

Directions

1. In a medium saucepan, combine the berries and maple syrup and bring to a simmer over medium to high heat, stirring frequently. Reduce the heat to medium-low and simmer for about 5 more minutes.
2. Stir in the chia seeds until thoroughly combined and cook, stirring frequently, until the mixture thickens to your desired consistency.
3. Let the jam cool in the pan for at least 15-20 minutes before putting it in the jar. It will thicken even more this way.
4. Once the jam is thick, remove the pan from the heat and stir in the vanilla. The jam should keep in an airtight container in the fridge for 1 to 2 weeks. It will thicken up a bit more when fully cooled.

Tip: Use grade B maple syrup which is usually the last taping from the tree and has the fullest flavor.

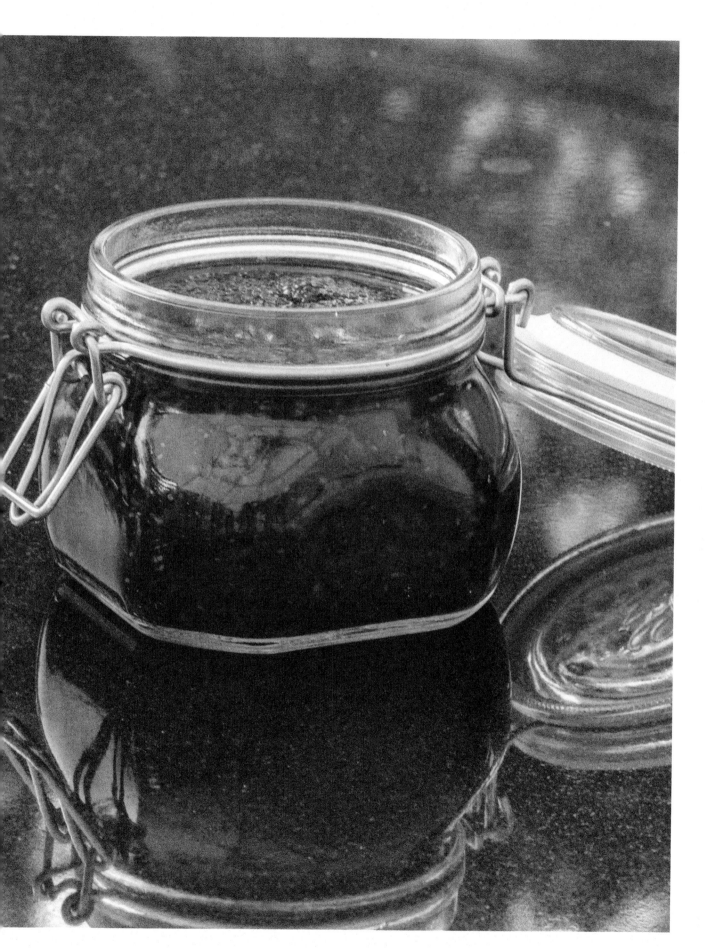

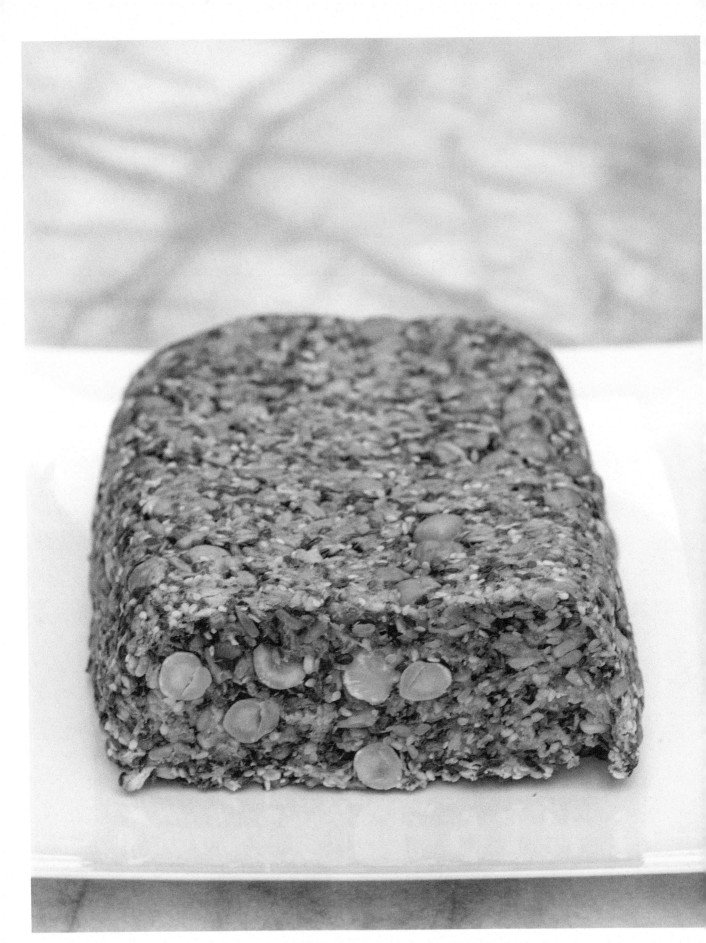

Hearty Gluten Free Nut, Seed and Oatmeal Bread

If you like a hearty slice of bread you will love this recipe! This whole-grain, gluten-free, no-knead, no-mess, life-changing loaf of bread is delicious. This recipe is adapted from My New Roots recipes.

75 minutes prep time with 2 hours rest time
makes 2 loaves

Ingredients

- 2 cups raw sunflower seeds not in the shell
- 1 cup whole flax seeds
- 1 cup blanched hazelnuts
- 3 cups rolled oats (if making gluten-free, make sure to get certified gluten-free oats)
- 4 tablespoons chia seeds
- 6 tablespoons psyllium husks
- Pinch of fresh ground coarse salt
- 2 tablespoons maple syrup
- 6 tablespoons coconut oil, liquefied at low temperature in a small pan
- 3 cups water

Directions

1. Place all dry ingredients in a large mixing bowl and combine well.
2. Whisk maple syrup, oil and water together in a small bowl.
3. Add this to the dry ingredients and mix very well until everything is completely soaked and dough becomes very thick (if the dough is too thick to stir, add one or two teaspoons of water until the dough is manageable). Smooth out the top with the back of a spoon.
4. Place the "batter" in two parchment lined loaf pans.
5. Let the pans sit out on the counter for at least 2 hours. To ensure the dough is ready, it should retain its shape even when you pull the sides of the loaf pan away from it or lift the parchment.
6. Preheat oven to 350° F.
7. Place loaf pan in the oven on the middle rack and bake for 20 minutes. Remove bread from loaf pan, place it upside down directly on the rack and bake for another 30 to 40 minutes. Bread is done when it sounds hollow when tapped. Let cool completely before slicing.

Tip: Store bread in a tightly sealed container for up to five days. It freezes well too, slice before freezing for quick and easy toast!

Caramelized Onion Hummus

Use as a base for wraps or for snacking with whole grain crackers or romaine lettuce.

15 minutes prep time
makes 2 cups

Ingredients

- 1 can chickpeas, drained and rinsed
- 2 tablespoons lemon juice
- 1 clove garlic minced
- ½ teaspoon salt
- ½ small white onion, sliced thin
- ½ teaspoon olive oil (optional)
- ¼ cup white balsamic vinegar
- 2 tablespoon date sugar
- fresh ground black pepper to taste
- smoked paprika for garnish

Directions

1. Sauté the onion until softened for about 5 minutes. You can sauté in ½ teaspoon olive oil or sauté without oil at all.
2. Add vinegar and date sugar and stir to combine with the onions. Continue to heat for about 5-7 minutes until the vinegar is reduced. Sprinkle with fresh ground black pepper and set aside.
3. Place onion mixture, chickpeas, garlic, salt and lemon juice into a food processor and mix until a smooth puree is formed.
4. Spoon into a covered container and refrigerate until ready to use. Top with paprika for a garnish.

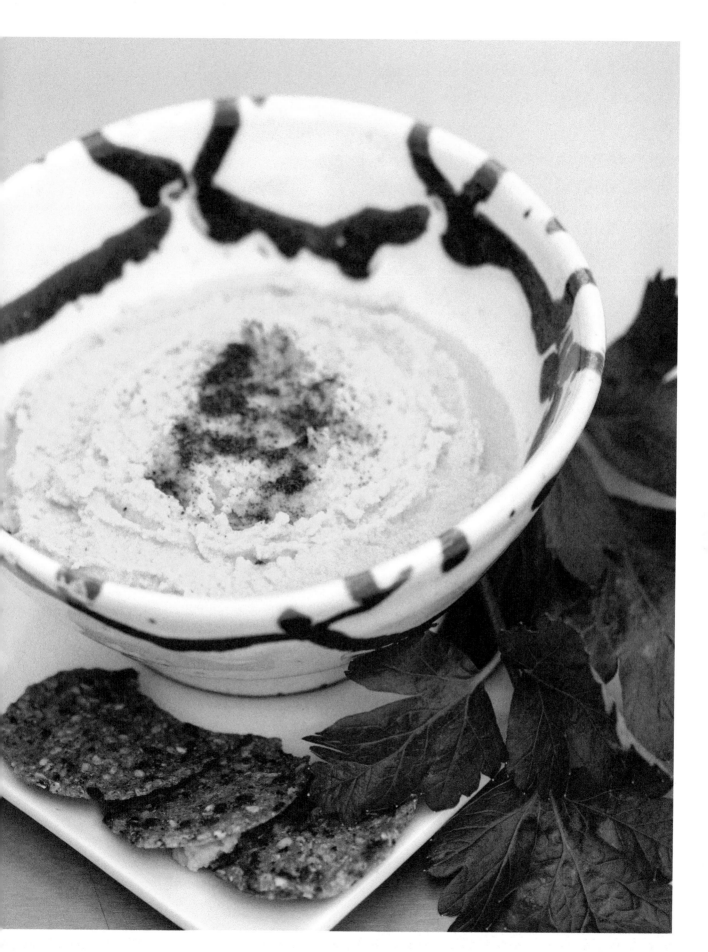

Almond Milk

Making almond milk is not only simple and quick but is a great substitution for cow's milk. It's rich and creamy and keeps in the refrigerator for 2-3 days. Using store bought blanched almonds eliminates the need for soaking and removing the skins.

3 minutes prep time
makes 4 cups

Ingredients

- 1 cup blanched almonds
- 4 cups cold water

Directions

1. Place the almonds and water in a high speed blender (I use a Vita Mix) and blend until smooth and creamy. Start out on a lower speed and gradually increase to high speed.
2. Be sure to blend long enough to get a smooth creamy texture. If processing is not completed long enough the milk will have a grainy texture. Substitutions using other nuts, such as raw cashews, can be used as well.

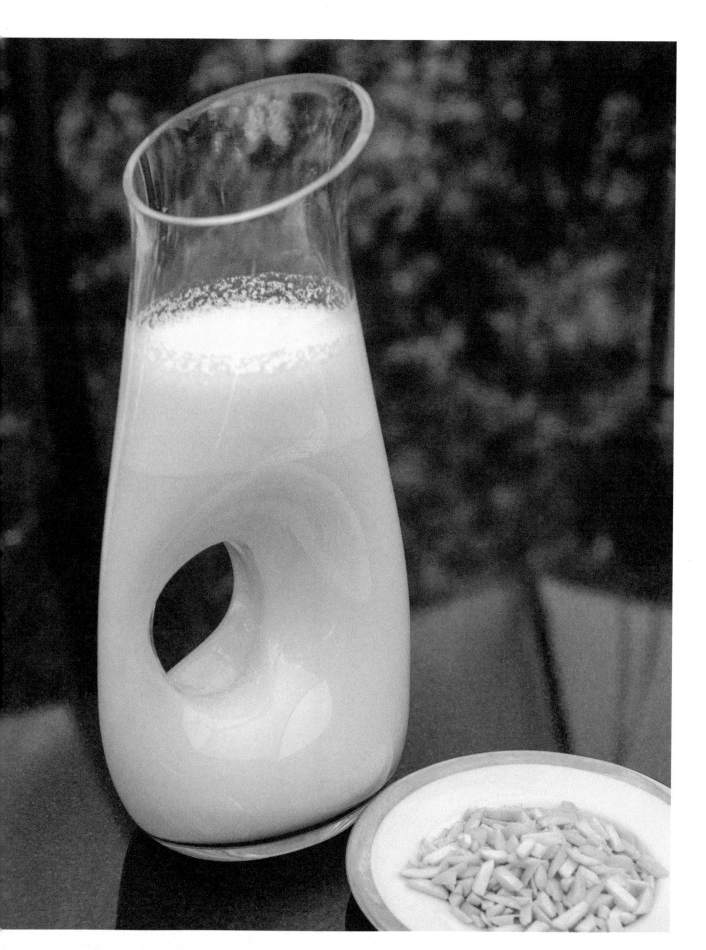

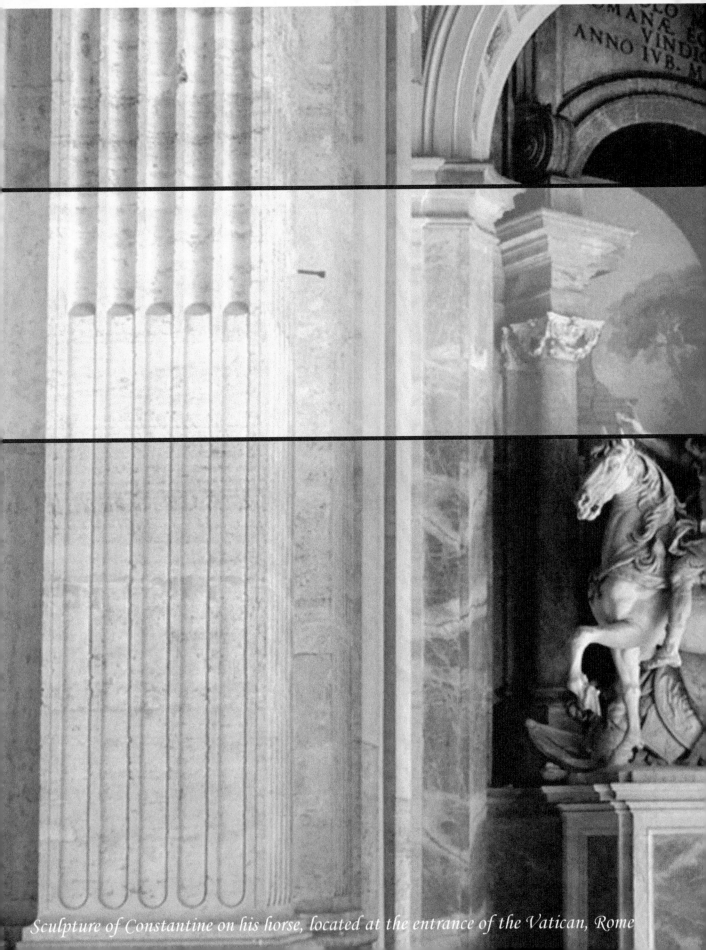

Sculpture of Constantine on his horse, located at the entrance of the Vatican, Rome

Chapter 9
Final Thoughts

One of the most gratifying things about the work I do is witnessing the transformation that takes place when high nutrient and fiber rich food replaces low nutrient, animal based products and processed foods. The results are nothing short of miraculous when the body receives what it needs to function optimally. In fact, compelling research indicates that a whole food plant based diet may likely reduce or eliminate reliance on a variety of medications.

At this point in my career I've seen hundreds of people who are genuinely interested in "eating cleaner." That is, by which I mean eliminating processed, sweetened and animal based foods and replacing them with more fruits and vegetables, nuts, seeds beans and legumes – preferably organically grown. Unfortunately, sometimes despite initial enthusiasm and absolute understanding of what is possible, even those deeply committed individuals can become derailed, falter and sometimes return to old habits.

While I was initially perplexed as to why and how this might happen, my experience now permits me to provide some insights which may give you a better understanding of potential pitfalls.

First, be careful not to fall prey to the "wizardry of marketing." Many times our food purchases are influenced by marketing and advertising and we end up buying (and eating) highly processed and unhealthful foods that are sold as a healthful product. For example, vegetable chips with a huge photo of a sweet potato on the front of the package is not the same as eating a real sweet potato. Similarly, "chicken breast" made from processed wheat and artificial chicken flavoring might seem like a plant based food, but it's highly processed and filled with artificial ingredients. This type of highly processed, low fiber and low nutrient food leaves one hungry and craving for more of the same, causing a never ending cycle of "self-medication." The resulting glucose and hormonal spikes and lows always seem to persist until dietary changes to whole, unprocessed foods, occurs.

The bottom line is this, try to buy only foods that do not have a label. Fruits, vegetables, whole grains, nuts and seeds do not require ingredient labeling because it's just the real thing - unaltered and nutrient dense just as intended.

When shopping, remember that healthful plant based eating strives to exclude foods with added sugar, salt and oils. Potato chips may be considered "plant based" but are not healthful food. The same goes for bakery and bread items. Stick with "real food for healthy people."

A concern I often hear about a plant based eating is that it may not provide enough protein. Somehow it seems this question always pops up and even if you're not concerned about it, others will ask "where are you getting your protein?" The reality is Americans get too much protein from animal sources. Beans, legumes and vegetables contain high quality protein. This topic could fill another book, however if this is a concern for you there is a much information available online about the protein content of all foods. You may find it interesting that I have not yet met a physician who has treated a patient for protein deficiency in the U.S. and neither have I. When I'm asked where I get my protein my response is this; "I'll tell you where I'm getting my protein if you tell me where you are getting your antioxidants, fiber and micronutrients;" invariably silence follows my question.

Understandably, clients become bored by eating the same meals over and over. This need not be the case. Options for delicious and satisfying plant based meals are unlimited. However, it takes a little time to develop a broad selection of great meals that you can enjoy. If you have read through or tried some of the recipes in this book I hope you will agree that eating plant based is not about deprivation, but about waking up your palate to foods that are nourishing and delicious. Don't be afraid to experiment in the kitchen! There likely will be times when a recipe doesn't turn out as you hoped. Remember, it's a learning experience and not a failure.

Without a doubt, acquiring new behaviors can be difficult to maintain. One of the best ways to stay on track is to build a support system by becoming part of a community of like-minded persons. Meet up and social groups can be found everywhere and are usually without cost to join. However, if there is not a viable group for you to join

in your area why not start one? When I began this journey several years ago, feeling alone, I started a meet up group with only myself as its first member. Although it started small it has grown to a large group that meets once a month. Our meetings focus on education, support and sharing of ideas

Last, while the field of nutrition has exploded with knowledge over the past 5 decades and it seems to remain in constant flux. Although what we hear almost every day may appear to be a contradictory series of findings, the following basic truth prevails. When we reconnect with real food and eliminate low nutrient, animal, processed, sweetened and low fiber foods, the body can and will heal itself in many ways. Research over and over confirms this very fact.

It's no secret that leaving our gardens and our kitchens separates us from the source of our food. Restoring this important connection allows us to truly nourish ourselves and to move closer to the gift of good health. I wish you well on the journey!

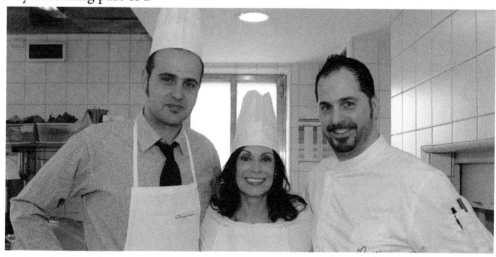

Testimonials

"Thank you so much for creating this class for us. It was such a wonderful experience in every way! It was hard to leave your beautiful home. We truly felt like we were on a short vacation."

— *Betsy R.*

"In every way a fantastic afternoon class - Great learning, fantastic food and the best company one could ever hope for!"

— *Joan L.*

"Her presentation was powerful enough to change the diets lifestyles of several of the firemen."

— *Dan Pease, Fire Chief, Highland Park, IL*

"Carol has done cooking demonstration at the Hospital for my patients. The food is fabulous and many of my patients have moved toward complete adoption of this approach after having attended Carol's inspiring workshops."

— *Dr. Kevin Fullin, cardiologist, United Health Systems*

"Your classes are a wonderful experience not only for the knowledge learned and delicious food but for the ambiance."

—*Beth D.*

"You are exceptional to work with. Your presentation and the dishes were delightful. I have already received lots of wonderful feedback from the patients who attended. I believe I knew nearly all of them personally. This was of tremendous help to them as these high risk patients continue to journey to recovery. Thank you so much."

— *Dr. Kevin Fullin, cardiologist, United Health Systems*

"I think your ears are ringing! I haven't stopped talking about my experience at Villa D'Anca. You are a delight! I learned a lot and enjoyed everything you shared with us."

— *Claudia L.*

"Never fails, you give an amazing event. Can I just say, we thoroughly enjoyed it, our stomachs mostly. The time flew, we were having so much fun. I loved the people there, I think we could become friends. I am thankful for the world you have opened up to us. Not only introducing us to some very nice people, but, also making us aware of the endless possibilities of obtaining a healthy lifestyle."

— *Sylvia C.*

"It is a long trip driving by myself.---but I love coming and learning. Thank you again Carol for your time and efforts. You have changed lives! I appreciate you!"

— *Terrie H.*

"Thank you again for such a wonderful class yesterday! It is always so refreshing to hear confirmation and see you in action with your recipes. So inspiring :-)"

— *Monica S.*

"I enjoyed it very much! It was not just a cooking class. It was an experience! Carol just keeps making things better and better!"

— *Terrie S.*

"Thank you for a lovely afternoon. I enjoyed meeting you and appreciate what you taught and prepared in your beautiful home. Having lunch in your backyard did feel like a leisurely eating experience with family and friends....food, wine, conversation."

— *Myra D.*

"Carol, it was a totally EXQUISITE day!"

— *Joan L.*

"I think I speak for everyone who attended your workshop when I say it was a fabulous program. I learned a lot and I'm very motivated to eat healthier and try new things."

— *Chris P.*

"I hope you will continue doing this great service. You give it your all and a little bit more and are so talented. You have so much to share with the world and know how to bring people together."

— *Wendy B.*

"I saw many people who had advanced heart disease and I was so frustrated because I knew if they just knew how to do the right thing, simple lifestyle and diet steps, that the entire trajectory of their life and health would have been different."

— *Dr. Mehmet Oz*

I am grateful to everyone who helped create this book.

My husband, Giovanni D'Anca: For your patience while I was compiling and completing this book, for your expertise when I needed help to find just the right words, for your support and encouragement, and most recently, for the gift of your photography that has made this book a work of art in addition to it becoming a manual for others needing guidance in their journey to better health. Your inspiration, love and support have played a huge role in making this book possible.

My parents: for the gift of raising me in a rich and meaningful culture that provided the basis for my love of cooking, community and a lifestyle that promotes longevity, and for my daughters who early on, by their very existence, have enriched my life beyond what I could have imagined. I am thankful.

My editor: Rachel Cooper who stayed the course, and for the work it took to make this book all that it could be. Your technical skills have made this book come alive.

To Terri Bold: for her assistance on hot summer days making recipes in my kitchen and assisting in many ways.

To: Taral Patel for applying his extraordinary technical and creative skills to the manuscript and for his wonderfully consistent support. I am grateful.

To: Mark Lieberman and Bob Kaden for your encouragement, guidance and support when I was considering writing this book.

To: Dr. Kevin Fullin for your bold courage to want something more for your patients through offering education for preventing, and at times, reversing chronic illness through nutritional intervention, and for the example you set each and every day in the care that you take with your patients.

To: Dr. Stephen Devries for the hours spent discussing nutrition in minute detail as it relates to better outcomes for patients. For your support of the work that I do, for all your encouragement and for helping me better define my path. Your leadership at the Gaples Institute inspires me.

To: Joan Levin, a constant supporter of my work, for the example you provide and for showing us what is possible when legislative changes are needed to protect the health of our nation.

To: Dr. Neal Barnard for your comments at the end of this book and for your national leadership with plant based nutrition.

To: All of my "Academy of Plant Based Nutrition" students and my clients whether past or present. Working with you has helped me grow in the knowledge of what is needed most to help others. I've learned as much from you as you have learned from me and I am grateful.

To: My entire meet up members whether past or present. Your presence at our monthly meetings is inspiring and your questions push me in the quest for more in the never ending pursuit of nutritional knowledge.

Index

CPSIA information can be obtained
at www.ICGtesting.com
Printed in the USA
BVOW10s1545160316

439869BV00012B/11/P